A Guide on how to Prepare for your New-born Baby. Proper Feeding, Sleeping, and Care

Copyright 2018 by Joseph R. Parker- All rights reserved.

This document is geared towards providing exact and reliable information in regards to the topic and issue covered. The publication is sold with the idea that the publisher is not required to render accounting, officially permitted, or otherwise, qualified services. If advice is necessary, legal or professional, a practiced individual in the profession should be ordered.

- From a Declaration of Principles which was accepted and approved equally by a Committee of the American Bar Association and a Committee of Publishers and Associations.

In no way is it legal to reproduce, duplicate, or transmit any part of this document in either electronic means or in printed format. Recording of this publication is strictly prohibited and any storage of this document is not allowed unless with written permission from the publisher. All rights reserved.

The information provided herein is stated to be truthful and consistent, in that any liability, in terms of inattention or otherwise, by any usage or abuse of any policies, processes, or directions contained within is the solitary and utter responsibility of the recipient reader. Under no circumstances will any legal responsibility or blame be held against the publisher for any reparation, damages, or monetary loss due to the information herein, either directly or indirectly.

Respective authors own all copyrights not held by the publisher.

The information herein is offered for informational purposes solely, and is universal as so. The presentation of the information is without contract or any type of guarantee assurance.

The trademarks that are used are without any consent, and the publication of the trademark is without permission or backing by the trademark owner. All trademarks and brands within this book are for clarifying purposes only and are the owned by the owners themselves, not affiliated with this document.

Contents

Introduction 1

Chapter 1: The first days 4

Chapter 2: Your baby's breathing 30

Chapter 3: Feeding your new-born 37

Chapter 4: New-born and baby hygiene 57

Chapter 5: Why do babies cry a lot? 69

Chapter 6: Your baby's senses 78

Chapter 7: Development and growth 86

Conclusion 96

Introduction 108

Chapter 1: The first day at home with your baby 111

Chapter 2: All about baby sleep 138

Chapter 3: Dealing with separation anxiety 156

Chapter 4: How to properly feed your baby 164

Chapter 5: Your baby's development 185

Conclusion 198

Introduction

There's nothing quite like a baby's first months of life, as they are arguably the ones that will have the most impact throughout the first stages of their development: their overall health, mood and energy are all greatly impacted. It's normal for infants to double in weight during the first 5 months of their lives, and by their first year, even their brain size has increased by thirty percent. Who else but a baby is able to grow over 10 inches in a year?

If you're a first-time parent, you're probably starting to feel stressed out about all the things you'd need to do in order to make all of this growth and development happen. The good news for parents is that nature pretty much takes care of things and that it's not necessary to do that much, as the transitions a baby goes through seem to occur almost on schedule.

Unlike pretty much everything else today, babies don't come with instruction manuals. In fact, no one knows how to raise children by the book because such a book does not—neither will it possibly ever—exist.

This book does not claim to contain all the information that parents will ever need. Rather, its main goal is to simply steer parents in the right direction as far as raising a baby is concerned. There is no one-size-fits-all solution when it comes to raising children because they all have very different needs and personalities. Hence, this book was written in the hope of serving as a basic guide for parents regardless of what makes their newborn unique.

Whether you are a first-time parent or a veteran currently waiting for your fourth one, I hope that the advice in this book helps make life a just a bit easier for you and your new family member.

Chapter 1: The first days

When you see your new-born for the first time, you might feel a wide range of different emotions that could go from complete exhaustion to total joy. If this is your first baby, it might even feel a bit odd to be home for the first time with him. You might be overwhelmed with thoughts about how your life will be altered forever. What was previously an adult home prior to this event, is now officially your new family home, thanks to the little one you've now brought to this world.

Even if you did your best to be well prepared for your baby's arrival by buying all the important stuff and constantly thinking about what life as a parent would be like, there's lots of adjustments to be made. For some parents, the whole thing might even feel a bit anticlimactic.

New parents tend to get too stressed about how their new baby is doing and will spend hours watching him to make sure that things such as his breathing and movements are normal. You might even forget about the difference between night-time and daytime for a while. A lot of your focus will be on making sure that your new-born's needs are being met, and that's a 24 hour job in the earliest stages.

You might have fallen in love with your child from the first you saw him, but it's completely normal if you need some time to build attachment and start feeling a connection. Some parents are completely exhausted after their baby's birth to be able to bond with him immediately. In some other instances, a mother's feelings tends to get affected by things such as having had a long labor or a complicated birth.

Take your time but try to have as much contact with your new-born as possible. Although your new-born has very poor eyesight, he has a great sense of smell and touch and will enjoy snuggling and bonding with his parents.

In some instances, depending on the conditions of how the birth went, the midwife could give you a visit home at some point during the first days to check that everything's fine with the baby and his mother.

How a mother's body changes after birth

Your body has done the incredible job of bringing new life into our world. It's perfectly normal to feel exhausted, sore and even a bit sad. Over the next days, there will be a few changes that your body will go through. There's no way around this regardless of how you gave birth and whether you've chosen to breastfeed or formula feed your baby.

Soon after birth, mothers experience bleeding that initially resembles a heavy period. This bleeding usually decreases after 2-6 weeks. You'll need to wear a sanitary towel during this stage.

A lot of women experience constipation after they give birth. To make things easier for you, try eating high-fibre foods, and stay well hydrated. If things don't improve, you can ask your doctor to recommend a laxative or stool softener.

In some instances, there can be complications after birth and there are some signs and symptoms that you should be watching out for. The main ones are:

- Postpartum haemorrhage: losing 500ml of blood or more in a short period of time. This usually happens while the mother is at the hospital, so it's easy to receive treatment immediately. If you're at home and you start bleeding heavily, don't hesitate to call an ambulance.

- Severe and persistent headaches: this could be a sign of pre-eclampsia, which is usually accompanied by vision problems, nausea, vomiting and heartburn.

- High fever: This can be a sign of an infection that spread from one part of your body to another.

- Abdominal pain: If you feel sick and start feeling pain in the upper part of your abdomen or upper right side of it, it might be a sign of a rare condition that affects how the liver works and how your blod cloots.

If you ever notice any of these or any other abnormal symptoms, act quickly and call your doctor as soon as possible. These can all be very serious and have life threatening consequences if not treated properly.

Your body is coping with fluctuating hormonal levels and is seriously sleep-deprived, while your mind is trying to adjust to this new chapter of your life. The discomforts you're feeling are normal, because you've gone through an incredible nine-month journey, and it's important to give yourself enough time and care need to recover fully.

How the breasts change after starting breastfeeding.

If you are breastfeeding, your will produce colostrum, which precedes regular milk. Colostrum is full of antibodies and provides your child with a protein boost and gives support to his immune system. It will take a few days for regular milk to come in, and it could take a while more if you gave birth by c-section. When your breasts are getting ready for regular milk production, you'll notice that they become significantly fuller and firmer.

Lots of people think that regular milk production starts naturally, but it's normal to hit a few bumps, especially first time moms at the early stages. Even though your midwife might have shown you the proper way how to breastfeed while you were at the hospital, you might have a hard time once you're at home with your newborn.

It can be tricky to get a proper latch going, and be able to breastfeed for extended periods of time. Many mothers will get sore nipples at first. Try different positions to avoid cracking and discomfort.

When breastfeeding, it doesn't matter whether you're sitting, lying back or the place you do it. What you should be focusing on is making sure that you feel comfortable and that your baby can latch properly without much trouble.

-To start, choose either to lie or sit on your back so that it is well supported and there's no discomfort.

-If necessary, raise your feet or knees.

-In case you are sitting up, a pillow can be a great support, as it will take weight of your baby so that your forearms don't get tired.

-If you're laying back, cushions and pillows can be used to support the back and shoulders. Once you feel at ease, put your baby's abdomen down on your chest and tummy, so that he has somewhere to push on with his feet. Your body will give him enough support and help him make adjustments to get a proper latch.

- If you choose to lie on your side, lay your baby alongside with you and place his tummy towards yours.

You can try other positions such as:

- The cradle hold, where you place your baby's head in the crook of your arm.

- The rugby ball hold, where you place your baby's body under your arm.

- Laid-back, where you're lie back, supported by cushions or pillows.

Don't be afraid to experiment a bit to find the position that is most comfortable for you and your baby.

Getting a proper latch

-Your baby has to use his tongue and bottom lip to get to your breast, and should touch it as far away from the nipple's base as possible.

-Bring your child to your breast so that his head faces your nipple and doesn't have to exert extra effort to turn his head to find and reach it. Make sure that the nose is in line with your nipple. This will give him enough room to tip his head back prior to latching on. Your baby's chin should be leading and his mouth should be open so that his lips touch your nipple.

-Your baby's natural response should be to drop his lower jaw. Now, depending on your position, you may be able to help him adjust and get his lower lip as far away from your nipple's base as possible. If you're in a laid back position, his natural reflexes should help guide him and root for your nipple.

-Your baby's reflex response can be triggered by brushing the mouth with your nipple. By using his sense of touch, your baby will find your breast.

Quick tips to make breastfeeding flow smoothly.

-The forearm is a much better support for the baby's shoulders than the wrist.

-Place the palm of your hand behind your child's shoulders and the index finger and thumb behind the ears.

-Gently cradle your child's head using your whole hand, so that he can still move it. You can also use your hand to guide and help him get a good latch.

-If you are having a hard time keeping the baby's hands out of your way, you could try wrapping him in a soft blanket.

Using nipple cream after breastfeeding can help relief some of the initial discomfort and prevent cracking. Most creams don't need to be removed before the next feeding session. Your own milk can also be used as a nipple moisturizer. But remember that breastfeeding shouldn't be painful. If your nipples are getting sore after the initial adjustment period, it's usually a sign that your baby isn't latching on correctly.

What happens when you choose to formula-feed your baby?

If you've chosen to feed your child with formula, talk to your midwife or breastfeeding counsellor about the best way to suppress milk production. The body has begun the milk production process, and it'll need some time to shut down again.

Whenever the milk production process starts, you'll notice that your breasts will look much fuller than before. The engorgement initially causes some discomfort, but it soon tapers off after the first week.

To handle the temporary discomfort, you can ask your doctor for pain relievers or if mild, you may use ice packs and special bras for support. In some cases, the engorgement might feel a bit overwhelming, and you may need to express some of your milk by hand to feel less discomfort.

How your body feels after a vaginal birth

If you've had a vaginal birth, you're probably experiencing some soreness. In case you had a tear or an episiotomy, it could even be painful for a few days. Ice packs can help reduce some of the swelling. After peeing, you may use warm water from a jug to clean the area instead of wiping with a paper, which can be uncomfortable at this point.

Do not worry if you leak, or lose the sensation when going to pee. This won't last long. The nerves that connect to your pelvic floor muscles got exhausted during your baby's birth.

Doing some pelvic floor exercises can help strengthen the pelvic floor muscles. Initially, you may probably not feel much when you do them, or you may not be able to perform more than a simple twitch of your pelvic muscles. Doing these everyday can make a big difference.

How your body feels after a caesarean birth.

A caesarean is considered a major abdominal surgery. If you've had one, you need others to help you doing almost everything for at least a week or two, and you should never pick up anything heavier than your newborn. Very gentle activity can help speed up the recovery process.

Just like any other surgery, moving a bit can help your circulation and prevent the formation of blood clots. Staying still for long periods of time is a big no-no, as the pain will probably worsen when you try to move again.

The doctor or midwife will remove the surgical dressing after at least a day has passed. You should be keeping a close watch for any signs of infection. Common red flags are blood or pus from the surgical incision, or unpleasant odors.

Why am I feeling sad an irritable after giving birth?

Returning home with a baby in your arms is a major life event, and you shouldn't expect to get used to the changes right away. New parents find that it takes anywhere from a few days to a few months to feel that things finally feel normal again. While you're navigating through this massive adjustment phase, do what you can do let go of any fixed ideas you might have of how you expected things to be, and try enjoy things the way they are.

The impact can be overwhelming for mothers, since there lots of different hormones surging through their bodies after giving birth. During the first few days, you might experience baby blues. This is extremely common, and over 50% percent of moms get the baby blues at one point or another. Fortunately, these feelings don't last long and usually fade away after a few days or weeks.

Never be shy about asking others for help at these first stages, and always have someone nearby to speak to. Ask friends and family to help with basic chores such as doing the groceries, cooking, washing, etc. If you wish to spend some time alone together with your baby, that's fine, too.

If you're still feeling happy and are having lots of negative thoughts, be on the lookout for signs of postnatal depression, which can have serious consequences and should be properly treated by a professional. Speak to your physician about how exactly you're feeling. Not treating postnatal depression affects not only you, but everyone around you, including your new baby.

Why am I peeing a lot after giving birth?

During pregnancy, your body stored a lot of fluid. Now that you've given birth, all of this fluid needs to go somewhere.

In the days following birth, it's very likely that you will be peeing for a lot more than what you're used to. This is the easiest way for your body to get rid of the extra fluid. You will also sweat more. You might want to clean or shower more frequently when you're dealing with this phase.

Due to so much fluid moving around, your feet and ankles may become swollen. The swelling may even be worse than what you had during pregnancy.

Even though your body is trying to get rid of extra fluid, it's very important to drink a lot of water to protect your bladder and kidneys. Being well hydrated may also help to avoid constipation.

If you are breastfeeding, you will be thirsty frequently due to the regular milk production that's going on. It's recommended to have a bottle of water around at all times. Avoid drinking too many sugary drinks.

Is it normal for pee to leak after coughing, sneezing or laughing?

After giving birth, it is very normal for pee to leak a bit after coughing, sneezing or exercising. This is known as stress incontinence.

The pelvic floor muscles stretch in the front to the rear of the pelvis, and behave like a supportive sling. These muscles play a key role in controlling bladder and bowel movements.

The body changes a great deal while pregnant, and as your child grows, he pushes both your bladder and urethra. Not only this, but the hormonal changes and the stress the body has gone through after labour all affect the function of your pelvic floor muscles. When these muscles aren't working properly, they may cause stress incontinence.

These changes, alongside hormone changes and also the stress of work, can all affect how good your pelvic floor muscles work. If they're no longer working well, stress incontinence can be the result.

The good news is that it's very easy to speed up the recovery process and strengthen these muscles again by performing pelvic floor exercises or Kegels. Kegels in particular can be very helpful as they can be performed anywhere, in almost any position.

Anywhere from 10-30 Kegels per day can be enough to strengthen back your pelvic floor muscles. To perform a Kegel repetition, imagine that you're trying to stop the flow of pee or the passing of gas. While performing these, avoid moving your legs, buttocks or tummy muscles. No one should be able to tell that you're performing these, and you can do them almost anywhere!

It's normal to not feel any improvements after a week or a few days following birth, because your nerves have been completely exhausted. But continue to do the exercises. After a few weeks, you'll start noticing the difference.

In some rare cases, mothers continue to have incontinence issues even after a few months have passed. If this is the case, or if on the other hand, you are having difficulty peeing, speak to your physician.

Is it normal to have stomach cramps after giving birth?

What you are feeling is the uterus going back and contracting to its normal, pre-pregnancy size. These cramps are known as "after-pains", and are usually felt 48 to 72 hours after giving birth.

These pains can be more intense if you've had twins or triplets, or are breastfeeding. Ibuprofen can be very helpful for easing the after pains and can be taken while you're breastfeeding.

Right before you gave birth, your womb was much bigger than it was before pregnancy. Sometimes up to 20 times bigger. After you give birth, your midwife should check your womb, either at your own home, or the hospital. Your physician or midwife should check your belly again after the usual six week postnatal check.

Why do I still look pregnant after giving birth?

The muscles at your tummy extended and weakened as the size of your baby increased. So, your belly might have a similar shape to what it was before pregnancy. Mothers often feel concerned about this, but it is completely normal, and the skin gets back to normal after a few weeks. Eating a healthy diet plan and being active once you're able to, helps speed up the recovery.

Some specific postnatal exercises can be excellent for getting back into shape and toning up. These may also help with backache. Ask your midwife or doctor about your options, as each case should be treated individually depending on the mother's condition.

Why can't I sit down comfortably?

Things such as an episiotomy or having a perineal tear can make it very difficult to sit down without feeling discomfort or pain. The tears usually happens when your vagina isn't able to stretch enough when giving birth. An episiotomy is a cut that the midwife or doctor makes in the perineum to help make the vagina opening bigger so that it's easier for the baby to come out.

The majority of the tears occur in the perineum, which is the space between the vagina and the anus. Tears can affect the skin, muscles and in some cases even the bowel. Most mothers that have had a vaginal birth will experience a tear at some point after birth.

Most tears tend to be small and heal on their own, while others are deeper and require stitches to heal correctly. Around 60 percent of women who tear will need to have stitches. Stitches are also necessary if you've had an episiotomy.

The stitches are going to be uncomfortable for a few weeks or days. Ask your doctor about which pain killers you're able to take at this point. Ice packs can help alleviate some of the discomfort in the area.

If you're not sure that you're healing properly, or if the pain doesn't get better or you notice any odd smells around the wound area, be sure to talk to your doctor or midwife about it.

Chapter 2: Your baby's breathing

Your baby has spent a lot of time covered in amniotic fluid inside his mother's womb, so there's a lot of new adjustments to be made now that he's outside at last.

New parents tend to react to every little thing that their newborn does, from hiccups, cries and odd sounds. Their reaction is normal and the great news is that all babies come with incredible instincts that help them cope with their new lives and environment.

These instincts will be there to signal others they're hungry or uncomfortable by crying. They also help babies want to be close to you. Try placing a finger in your baby's tiny palm and notice how he'll hold on to it.

I'm constantly worried about my new-born's breathing

First time parents usually stay awake during the first night at home with their baby just to make sure that he's breathing all right. The occasional snort, sneeze or odd sound is very normal for new-borns and there's usually nothing to be worried about.

Do not worry if you hear a few squeaks or snuffles here and there. A new-born has only recently started to inhale air for the first time and it's a very different process to what he was used to while inside his mother's belly. This new environment is very dry compared to where your baby was.

Your child is making little snorts and grunts because he's trying to breathe through the nose, which lets him feed and breath at the same time.

Babies are unable to blow their own noses, and because of this, mucus tends to stay and accumulate, creating whistles, sniffles or snorting sounds. When it goes back to your baby's throat, it may cause him to make gurgling sounds that can alarm some parents.

When the mucus travels more towards the larynx and trachea, your baby may sound a bit "chesty". If you lightly put your hands on top of your baby's chest, you might feel a gentle rattle, which is a vibration in the larynx. But this is nothing to be concerned about. Your baby's breathing might remain like this for a few days or weeks.

Your baby's breathing might even become irregular for some time, with a combination of quick breathing and slower breathing.

However, if you're very worried about your baby's breathing, don't be afraid to call your doctor or midwife. Midwives expect calls from new mothers at all times during the first days following birth.

Why do new-borns have hiccups?

Hiccups are normal and normally don't cause any discomfort. Babies usually experience hiccups for the first time while they're inside their mothers belly, so they are used to them. It's common for babies to have them or bring up a bit of their last feed.

Bringing up feed is caused by reflux. Reflux is caused when the muscular valve at the end of the food pipe (which helps keep the food inside the belly), needs more time to get stronger and be more efficient. This doesn't happen overnight and is a gradual process. As your baby grows and so does his stomach capacity, the food pipe should lengthen and your baby should stop having this issue often.

Particularly at this very early stage, your child may bring up amounts of milk that go from small to what may seem like their whole feed. Always keep a muslin or cleaning cloth nearby. Eventually, you'll develop a sense to what's normal and what's not. Just make sure to drape a cloth over your shoulder.

Should I burp my new-born?

It's probably not necessary to burp your child at this point. Your newborn's tummy is very small, usually the size of a marble. As mentioned before, during the first day, your breasts will produce colostrum to feed and nourish your baby with antibodies and nutrients.

If your baby is having a hard time feeding in the first days, you may need to express some of the colostrum yourself. When doing this, the amount might seem small, but this is very normal. With colostrum, a tiny bit goes a long way. Your child will drink as much as he needs. His feeding requirements will increase gradually once milk comes in, which usually happens after a few days, once your breasts stop producing colostrum.

Your child is only able to take in a tiny bit of colostrum at a time and might even need to take a few rests, as it takes a considerable amount of effort to use the mouth and jaw muscles. With these rest periods, you might find that your new-born's first feeds can take a while, sometimes up to 40 minutes or an hour, so make sure that you're in a comfy spot where you can relax and have something to eat and drink nearby if necessary.

While both you and your new-born get used to the feeding, little bubbles of air and milk might end up inside his belly. If you are formula-feeding your child, he's more prone to swallow air as he drinks from the bottle. Nevertheless, your child is going to be taking such small quantities of milk during the first days that it's unlikely he'll need to be burped.

Whenever your baby gets bubbles inside his tummy, he'll feel more comfortable if he burps to release them. Some babies can do this on their own and don't need any help, while others will appreciate if you lend them a hand.

Chapter 3: Feeding your new-born

Choosing between breastfeeding and formula feeding is one of the first decisions that parents make regarding how their newborn. Let's take a look at some nutrition guidelines so that you know what's right for you and your new baby.

Breast milk vs formula milk

Most paediatric institutions, including the American Academy of Paediatrics, recommends that babies should be breastfed if possible, during at least 6 months. Mothers may choose to continue breastfeeding beyond the first year if they want to.

However, breastfeeding isn't always possible or even preferable for all mothers. Choosing whether to breastfeed or not usually depends on the mother's comfort levels and her lifestyle. In some specific cases, breastfeeding might not be the ideal option for a mother and her baby.

Although breast milk is more nourishing to a baby, there are high quality formulas available, and his nutritional needs should be met regardless of which method you choose.

Breastfeeding

There are several advantages breastfeeding has over formulas. One of the most important is that breast milk is the ideal food for a new-born's digestive system. It includes all the important nutrients that a baby needs, and its main components (such as lactose and fat) are usually easily digested by babies. Formulas tend to do their best to imitate breast milk, and in many cases come close, but aren't able to match their exact composition.

Breast milk also has the advantage of including antibodies that do a great job at protecting babies from infections such as digestive or respiratory infections. Research has suggested that breastfed children are less prone to develop certain conditions such as diabetes, allergies and asthma. It also decreases the chance that the child becomes overweight later on.

Breastfeeding has benefits for mothers too. To produce milk, the body uses resources and burns calories as a result, so breastfeeding mothers are sometimes able to get back in shape faster. Research suggests that it also protects mothers from breast and ovarian cancer.

Some moms also find breastfeeding more practical than formula feeding, as it requires no preparation and you rarely run out of milk when feeding your child normally. Also, there are almost no extra expenses to make. Although nursing mothers have to eat a bit more and may want to buy certain accessories such as nursing bras or breast pumps, these expenses are little when compared to the costs of formula feeding over several months.

Another perk of breastfeeding is that it complements the emotional needs of babies and mothers, as the skin to skin contact helps with connection and bonding. Also, mothers that feel confident that they are giving their child all the nourishment they need can help them feel more confident in their parenting abilities.

Cons of Breastfeeding

After hearing so many positive things about breastfeeding, why is it that not every mom chooses to do it?

First of all, breastfeeding is a huge commitment, and some mothers might feel restricted by the demands of a nursing baby. Since breast milk can be easily digested, breastfed babies usually eat more often than formula fed babies. This means that the mom may find herself tied down to his child's demands often every 2-3 hours during the earliest stages. Initially, this can be very tiring, but babies eventually feed less often and sleep more during the night.

Some moms have responsibilities such as working outside home that makes it difficult for them to breastfeed. For these moms, formula feeding is a very practical solution, and even her partner or other caregivers can easily feed the baby with a bottle. Of course, mothers that wish to continue breastfeeding can always use a breast pump to collect milk so that the baby still gets it while mom is around. Other family members such as the father may want to share the responsibility of feeding the baby.

Sometimes, mothers feel embarrassed about breastfeeding around others. These feelings usually fade once the mother gets the hang of the breastfeeding process and feels more confident with it. It can sometimes be helpful to hear from other mothers that have nursed. Also, the majority of hospitals have staff that can give new mothers the necessary instructions on how to correctly breastfeed their baby before they go home.

In some instances, a mother's health may be preventing her to breastfeed. Examples of this are mothers that are undergoing chemotherapy or mothers with HIV. If you have any medical condition or take medicines on a regular basis, it's best to talk to your doctor and check if it's fine to breastfeed before starting. If your doctor tells you to stop breastfeeding temporarily, you can always continue pumping breast milk so that milk production continues.

In some cases, it's not possible to breastfeed the child, for example when the baby is ill or born prematurely. Moms should consult with their doctor's about expressing and storing their milk. Even if the baby can't be breastfed, milk can always be given through a tube or a bottle.

Mothers that have had plastic surgery done on their breasts or have inverted nipples, may run into problems when breastfeeding. But this can usually be overcome with the help of a lactation nurse.

Mothers that choose to nurse should avoid giving pacifiers or bottles to their babies, at least until breastfeeding becomes familiar after a few weeks. Introducing these before starting breastfeeding can confuse the child and lead to him eventually refusing his mother's breast.

Formula feeding

Commercially sold formula can be a good alternative to breast milk. Bottle feeding gives mothers a lot of freedom and makes it simple to measure how much food the baby is getting. Also, babies that are fed formula milk usually ask to be fed less often than those who breastfeed. This is because it takes longer for them to digest formula milk than breast milk.

With formula feeding, pretty much anyone can feed the baby at any time. There's no need for the mother to express milk from her breast if someone else will feed the baby. It can be a highly practical solution for mothers that lead busy lifestyles.

Cons of formula feeding

Similar to how breastfeeding has its own restrictions, so does formula feeding. Formula feeding needs planning and organization, especially if you intend to take your child out. Also, the costs could be high for some families.

You have to be aware of how much formula is left, and make sure that the bottles you'll be using to feed the baby are clean.

Here's a few guidelines for baby formula:

-When preparing the formula, be sure to follow the instructions on the label as closely as you can, unless your child's paediatrician has given you special instructions.

-Discard any formula that has been left out of the fridge for more than an hour. If your baby leaves any formula in the bottle after feeding, never use it for subsequent feedings.

-You can prepare formula beforehand and store it in the fridge for up to 24 hours. Before feeding your child, make sure that you have carefully warmed the bottles. It's not necessary to warm up the bottles, but babies often prefer it that way.

-Avoid warming formula in a microwave, as it usually heats the bottle unevenly and can easily burn your baby's mouth. The best way to warm it up is to hold it in running warm water.

Eating frequency

Newborns typically eat 8 to 12 times per day during their first weeks. Formula fed babies may feed a bit less than that. Initially, moms could try breastfeeding for ten to fifteen minutes on each breast, and then make time adjustments as necessary.

Breastfeeding should always be done on demand, when your baby asks for it. Typically, babies will ask to be fed every one to three hours. As babies get older, they will require less feedings and the time between each session will be longer. Make sure that you monitor the number of times your baby feeds, as it is not normal to go more than four to five hours without feeding.

Your baby is probably hungry if he does any of the following:

-Moves his head from side to side.

-Opens his mouth.

-Sticks out his tongue.

-Puts his hand inside his mouth.

-Makes puckering gestures.

-Cries.

At this point, it is not necessary to set a feeding schedule for your baby. Schedules can be very useful but they should come until later. New-borns know when they're hungry and are great at letting their parents know that they need to be fed. They will also tell you when they've had enough food. Keep an eye out for signs that your baby is full. If you notice that he has significantly slowed down when sucking from the breast or the bottle or is unlatching or turning away from it, then he's probably had enough.

As your baby grows, he'll eat more during each feeding session and will go for longer periods of time between feedings. There will be some occasions when your child will be hungrier than usual. This is normal, so just feed him on demand. Breastfeeding mothers sometimes worry that they won't be able to produce enough milk for their baby, but this is rare. When your child breastfeeds, he stimulates milk production, and the mother's supply of breast milk will adjust to his demands.

Is my baby eating enough?

Your baby should be checked by a paediatrician 2-3 days after he leaves the hospital. During this check-up, your baby will be examined from head to toes and it's a great moment to ask if he has any special feeding needs.

In most cases, you can be assured that your child is eating enough when he seems satisfied, wets his diapers anywhere from 5 to 8 times per day, poops regularly and is constantly gaining weight. On the other hand, if your baby seems irritable, cries a lot, and doesn't seem satisfied after a feeding session, then he might not be getting enough to eat. If you're worried that your child isn't getting enough food, call his paediatrician.

It's normal for babies to spit up small amounts of milk after eating, or while burping, but it's not normal for them to vomit. Vomiting can be a red flag for certain issues such as allergies or digestive problems.

Nutritional supplements for new-borns

Breast milk is very nourishing to babies and has the right amount of vitamins and iron. Healthy babies nursed by healthy moms don't need to take any additional supplements. The only exception is Vitamin D.

Most Paediatric Institutes recommend that nursing babies take vitamin D supplements until they start taking vitamin D fortified formula. Babies that are formula fed usually don't need to take supplements, as most formulas are usually fortified with enough vitamin D.

It's not necessary to give your baby water, juice, or other kinds of foods before the first six months. Breast and formula milk will provide everything they need.

Digestive problems

Your baby is bound to have a few minor digestive issues during the first days of his life, but these usually go away without any special attention. However, there are some cases where infections or congenital malformations can affect their digestive tract.

Here's a few of the most common digestive problems:

Spitting up. The majority of newborn babies are prone to spitting up either during their feeding session or afterwards. Some babies spit up with every feeding while others do so rarely. Another name for spitting up is gastroesophageal reflux, and it happens when the ring of muscle at the top part of the baby's stomach doesn't close correctly. Spit ups should decrease as your baby grows, and they usually go away completely by the time he reaches his first year.

There are a few ways you can help reduce your baby's spit up frequency or the amount being spit up.:

-Try feeding your baby before he's very hungry.

-Overfeeding tends to make things worse. If you're formula feeding your baby, try feeding him slightly smaller amounts.

-When formula feeding, check that the nipple isn't too large or small. When it is too large, milk usually flows to fast for the baby's stomach to handle. When it's too small, your baby will swallow lots of air.

-Avoid feeding your baby when he's distracted and keep feeding times when he's quiet and relaxed.

-Avoid putting tight clothing or diapers on your baby, as they can put unnecessary pressure on his tummy.

-Burping during the feedings and not only afterwards, can be a great way to get rid of excess air.

Spitting up is mostly harmless, however, when it happens often, it can lead to suboptimal weight gain and cause damage to the esophagus. If you notice any of the following signs, make sure to take your baby to the doctor:

-Persistent vomiting.

-Blood in the spit up.

-Your baby is not consistently gaining weight properly.

-The spit up causes your baby to gag.

Vomiting

While spitting up usually involves only small amounts of food, vomiting is stronger and can be a cause for concern when it's constant. Vomiting can signal that there's a viral infection in the digestive tract or an allergic reaction to something that your child ate.

To help your baby, try feeding him smaller amounts. It may be necessary to reduce the amount of time that your baby spends during each feeding session. To balance this, you should feed him more frequently.

Breast or formula milk might need to be replaced temporarily with an electrolyte solution. Before offering this, give your baby the solution at least eight hours after the last time he vomited. Start with small amounts and feed him frequently. 5 ml every five to ten minutes should be good to start. After 4 hours without vomiting, you can then double the amount you give him every hour. If your baby vomits again at some point, give his stomach a break for an hour and go back to feeding smaller amounts.

If your baby has a viral infection in his digestive tract, the vomiting is typically accompanied by diarrhoea. If you notice any green bile in his vomit, contact your doctor immediately. If your baby is vomiting and has diarrhoea, he will get dehydrated fast. If your baby is projectile vomiting, it could be a sign of a common condition in babies called pyloric stenosis. Surgery is typically required to correct this condition.

Sometimes, babies are born with digestive system abnormalities. These may form as a result of an issue with the baby's development during pregnancy. Although rare, these abnormalities have to be treated with surgery as early as possible.

These abnormalities can be found in the esophagus, stomach, abdominal wall, intestines or rectum.

Chapter 4: New-born and baby hygiene

Bringing your baby home for the first time is a very exciting moment for parents. It's also the time when your baby's body has to adapt to the challenges of the outside world.

When your baby has transitioned to his new environment, his immune system will be very underdeveloped and you'll need to help him fight off germs and diseases.

Here's a few tips to start off the right way:

Washing your hands

This sounds basic, but still extremely important. Germs are found all over your home and your hands. Washing with soap and water is one of the most efficient ways to avoid spreading germs and diseases. You can also use sanitizing towels or gel in case that there's no water and soap around.

Make sure that you wash your hands:

-Before feeding your baby, whether you're breastfeeding or formula feeding.

-After cleaning bodily fluids and substances such as poop, pee, vomit or saliva.

-If your hands look dirty.

-After using the bathroom.

As a new parent, you'll have your hands full of new responsibilities, and establishing hygiene routines at home can benefit everyone in your family. Surfaces and objects that are regularly touched should be cleaned often. Some of the most important are:

-Kitchen surfaces where you prepare food.

-Door handles around your house.

-Remote controls, switches.

-Mobile devices, computer keyboards.

-Bin lids.

Germs and infections from visitors

You're almost guaranteed to have family members and friends visiting you and your baby before expected. Don't be shy and always ask them if they've washed their hands before holding your baby. You should also ask them if they've been ill recently.

Vaccines

Vaccines are a very effective way to protect your child from infections and certain diseases such as polio and tetanus. Once vaccinated, your child's body will be more capable to fight off diseases.

Changing diapers

It's important to have good hygiene to prevent diaper rash and avoid spreading germs during diaper changes.

There are basically two kinds of diapers: disposable and reusable. Neither is better or worse for the environment, but they have each have their pros and cons and at the end, it mostly depends on each parents' lifestyle and their baby's.

Disposable diapers: Disposable diapers tend to be highly absorbent and are great at keeping your baby's skin dry and preventing rashes as a result. They're also very convenient, as all you have to do once they've been used is to throw them away in the garbage bin.

Reusable diapers: Although they tend to be less absorbent than disposable diapers, they are very cost effective since they can be re-used a lot. To avoid diaper rash, change them frequently.

It's also a good idea to have a changing mat that is comfortable for your baby so that the diaper changing process becomes a breeze. When buying a changing mat, choose one that can be easily washed and kept clean.

When changing your baby

-Unfasten the dirty diaper, hold your child's legs up by the ankles and remove the diaper. Make sure that it is well out of your baby's grasp.

-Cotton balls are very efficient at wiping your baby from front to back. Avoid wiping from back to front, as it can spread germs and cause infections, especially in girls.

-If your baby's a boy, he might pee after removing his soiled diapers from air exposure. Try placing a clean cloth or diaper over his penis soon as you remove the dirty diaper.

-It's best to fold the waistline of the diaper below the belly button area.

-Disinfect the changing mat or changing surface often.

-Always remember to wash your hands after each diaper change.

-Reusable diapers should never be washed alongside other clothing. Wash reusable diapers on their own, but remove any solid material in them beforehand by using a tissue. A hot wash works best for cleaning reusable diapers.

Dealing with diaper rash

Changing diapers will be a common thing now that your baby's home. There are several reasons why your baby might have diaper rash, most commonly: if their diapers are continuously wet, or if not changed often, diarrhoea and allergies. Certain laundry soaps can cause rashes. Keep an eye out for inflamed skin that has a bright red colour.

How to treat diaper rash

-Change your baby's diaper frequently and use a bigger size so that he can heal quicker.

-Thoroughly wash your baby with warm water after each diaper change. Do not use soap.

-Avoid rubbing your baby with the towel and gently pat him instead.

-Apply baby diaper cream or oil.

-Once your baby heals, consider continuing using the diaper cream or ointment to prevent rashes afterwards.

Bathing your new-born

It's not necessary to bath your new-born every day, and it is up to you to decide how often to wash him. As a general guideline, new-borns can be kept clean by bathing them two or three times per week. Bathing your baby can be a very fun and exciting ritual for you and your baby.

If you choose to bath your baby infrequently, you should always wash his face often, clean his genital and bottom after each diaper change and wipe grime and dirt off his skin.

Most babies love bathing and may even get excited about getting in the water. If you make it a fun routine, your baby will look forward to his bath time and there will be less crying and resistance. One of the most important thing to remember to make the process more pleasurable is to make sure that both the bathing area and the water at a warm temperature, because babies tend to lose heat from their bodies fast.

Sponge bathing

Sponge bathing is the best option until the umbilical cord stump heals. This usually takes around a week, but in some cases it may remain attached for up to two months.

Use a towel to wrap your child and keep him warm, and then uncover each area at a time to clean it with the sponge, water and a gentle baby wash.

-Clean your baby's face, and pay special attention to the hard to get spots such as creases behind the ears.

-Be careful with his eyes, and wipe them from the inside corner out. For this, it's best to use a piece of wool cotton.

-Clean his nostrils by using a wool cotton bud.

-The genital area is prone to infections when proper hygiene is not used. To prevent bacteria spreading there from the child's bottom, always clean from front to back.

Transitioning to tub bathing

Once your baby is three to eight weeks old, he's ready to transition to tub or bucket bathing. Keep in mind the following:

-Using more than two or three inches of water is unnecessary.

-Check that the water's temperature is just right before bathing your child.

-Your child's head, neck and shoulder area can be supported with your hand until they are able to sit straight.

-When the bathing is over, always clean and disinfect the area.

Chapter 5: Why do babies cry a lot?

Having your new-born home for the first time can be very exciting. However the realisation that you're responsible for him can be tough, especially when you hear him crying for the first time.

Whenever your baby cries, it doesn't always mean he's unhappy or uncomfortable about something. It's and instinctual response and the only method that your child knows at this point to get your attention - which he'll be using frequently!

How much do new-born babies usually cry?

You might be a bit surprised to hear that your first day at home with your baby is usually very quiet. Your child's body is getting used to the new environment and is recovering from the exhausting birth process.

In case your baby does cry early on, try to offer him your breast for comfort or the bottle if you are formula-feeding. While you're feeding your child throughout the day, soothe her by talking to him softly. Your voice and the sounds of your beating heart are very familiar to your baby, as he's used to hearing them while inside your belly.

Keeping your baby close to you will help you understand the cues he gives when hungry. Once you become better at noticing them, your baby won't need to cry too hard or too often to get your attention. If your baby is crying a lot, you might notice that it can be complicated for him to latch to your breast comfortably when feeding.

Your child may also be reassured by your scent, which he'll quickly recognize as her mother's. Fathers should also try to stay close to their new-born so that he quickly becomes familiar with his scent. Even though he has very poor eye sight, smell and touch are your newborn's most powerful senses. Holding your child in your arms will also be useful to nourish the bond between you.

Reasons for crying.

The number one reason for new-born cries is hunger. Your baby's marble sized tummy can't store much food for long which is why he'll have to breastfeed 2-3 hours to get the nutrients he needs to support all the growth he's doing. If you are formula-feeding your child, he might not be hungry if he's had milk in the past 2 hrs.

After a while, you'll have an easier time working out why your child is crying, and know what the best way to soothe him is. Here are a few other reasons why he might be crying:

Tiredness

Just like his parents, a child has gone through a very exhausting journey and might be feeling very tired. If too many visitors come to meet him, your baby can easily become over-stimulated. Do your best to have your baby in a relaxed environment so that he can rest and recover, so limit the amount of visitors if necessary.

He wants to be closer to you

Your child was as close as can be to you while inside your belly for nine months. Now he needs to face a totally "new world" full of sights, sounds, smells and textures. It's only natural for him to miss the comfort of his previous home. Notice if your baby stops crying when you give him a lot of close physical contact.

The temperature is not right

As the baby's skin gets used to his new environment, his body's temperature will have to adjust. A good rule of thumb is to use the same amount of layers as you'd wear plus one. If it's chilly, a soft blanket or a baby sleeping sack can warm him up.

Monitor your baby's temperature by touching his upper chest. If it's a bit too warm, remove a layer of clothing or a blanket, and add one in case it feels cold. It's not a good idea to check your baby's body's temperature by feeling his hands. It's normal for most babies to have hands and feet that are a bit cold to the touch. His hands might even have a bit of a blue colour, especially in the first days.

He needs a diaper change

Your baby will quickly notice when he has a wet diaper that needs to be changed. Some babies don't mind too much, while others that have sensitive skin do.

You might even notice that your baby cries while you're changing his diapers and it may be due to the cold air touching his skin while he's naked and wet. After a few days, you'll most likely be able to change him very quickly and the crying will diminish. If not, you can always talk, sing to your baby or use a toy to distract him during the change.

He doesn't feel well

Sometimes, crying can be one of the best ways for parents to realize that their baby isn't feeling well. Whenever you notice that your baby is crying in a different tone from the usual one, you should keep a close eye on him and try to determine the cause. You might notice that the crying is different if it's being weaker, higher pitched, or if it sounds more urgent.

Later on, teething might also cause some discomfort to your baby and cause him to be irritable and restless.

If your child is crying persistently and has a fever, diarrhoea or is vomiting, call your doctor right away.

He simply feels like crying

During the early stages, when your baby is less than 3-4 months old, you might notice that he usually cries more during the evenings. This is typical. Persistent crying in healthy babies is sometimes called colic. Your baby may feel a bit frustrated and refuse his parents efforts to comfort him. He may even clench his little fists and draw up his knees while he cries.

Some researchers had associated colic with tummy issues, perhaps caused due to intolerance to certain substances in the breast or formula milk, but nowadays, we have a better understanding of this very normal pattern of crying, and sometimes patience is the best ally you can have.

If the first day goes by and you manage to get through it without him crying, realize that it's very unlikely for him remain that way. During the next weeks, your baby will probably cry often during late afternoons and nights.

Most experts agree that as long as their health is in check, crying hard and long is a normal phase that babies go through. Even so, this can be very stressful for new parents.

You might not be able to always understand why your baby is crying accurately, and you might feel stressed of incompetent at times. Remember that this is very normal and it should fade once you understand your baby's cues and determine quickly what it is he needs.

Chapter 6: Your baby's senses

Your new-born may appear to do little more than eat, sleep, cry, pee, and poop during the day. However if you take a closer look at how your baby reacts to such things as light, noise, and touch, you will notice how his senses work at this early stage.

How your new-born sees the world

Newborns tend to see things best when they are eight to twelve inches away from their faces. Coincidentally, this is the perfect distance for gazing at his parents' faces (something that he will be doing very often). Any further than that, and your baby will see mostly fuzzy shapes because he is near-sighted. At birth, it is normal for a baby's eyesight to be between 20/200 and 20/400.

At this point, your baby's tiny eyes are too sensitive to vibrant lights, so they are more prone to open them when the lights are low. There's no need to worry if you notice that your newborn's eyes sometimes seem to be crossed or drift outwards, this is perfectly normal and will improve when his eyesight gets better and the eyes muscles become stronger.

Stimulate your baby's eyesight by giving him interesting things to look at. Babies tend to find human faces very interesting, but will also be curious about objects with bright colours and contrasting patterns. Things with movement are also very interesting to your baby. Interestingly, new-borns tend to find black and white objects more interesting than objects with lots of similar colours.

When quiet and alert, the typical new-born is able to follow the slow movements of human faces or objects.

Your baby's sense of hearing

Hearing is not new to your baby. He has been hearing sounds since he was inside his mother's belly. He got used to hearing mother's heartbeat, the sounds of her digestive system, and even the sound of her voice and those that she interacted with on a daily basis before he was born.

Once your baby is outside her mother's womb, he'll be hearing most sounds loud and clear. Just as he may be startled by unexpected sounds such as alarms or noisy motorcycles, he can be soothed by gentle sounds such as the voice of his parents or relaxing music.

Notice how he reacts to the sound of your voice. For your baby, his parent's voice tops the list of his favourite sounds. It's only natural, as he is aware that there is were warmth, care and food comes from. If your child is crying while in his crib, notice how quickly your voice may calm him down. Notice how your baby is able to listen to you while you're talking or singing in a gentle tone.

It's typical for babies to have a hearing screening at the hospital before they are sent home. It's even a requirement in most states. If your baby's hearing wasn't checked or if he was born at home or a special birthing center, he should still have a screening done before his first month of age. It's easy to diagnose hearing problems with this screening.

What about my baby's sense of taste and smell?

Newborns do have a sense of taste and will even have a preference for sweet tastes above all others. For instance, a new-born will have no problem sucking on a bottle of a sweet liquid, but will cry after he's given something sour or bitter. Similarly, babies will react positively toward smells they like and turn away from unpleasant smells.

Though at first, sweetness is preferred, your baby's preferences will develop throughout his first year. Studies have confirmed that a mother's diet can have a big impact on the way her milk tastes. Interestingly, these flavours can help shape your baby's taste preferences later in life, even throughout adulthood. For instance, a mother who ate lots of spicy foods while breastfeeding is more likely to have a child that prefers spicy foods later on.

The importance of touch

The sense of touch is extremely important to a newborn. He learns a lot of things about his new life out of the womb by touching.

While inside the mother's belly, babies are naturally kept warm and protected, but when outside, they have to face the feeling of cold, and new textures that may seem strange and uncomfortable at first, such as his crib, or stiff clothes. Make sure that you make things easier for him by providing soft clothes and blankets, and giving him lots of comfortable hugs, kisses and gentle touches.

If you are feeling worried

It's normal to be worried about your baby's senses and overall development. If you want some reassurance that everything is working well, you can do a bit of testing yourself.

When your baby is undistracted and in a quiet environment while he's active, do his eyes seem to cross more than just briefly? If so, it would be a good idea to call a doctor. Also do so if you notice that his eyes seem to be doing odd movements, or if they appear hazy or filmy.

It's common for newborns to be startled by loud noises nearby. You can check if your baby is hearing well by noticing if he calms down with the sound of your voice or if he responds to the sounds of a rattle. You can also experiment with music and see if he reacts.

Even when newborns pass the hearing screen at the hospital, you can always talk to your doctor if you're worried about your baby's hearing. The sooner potential problems are noticed, the better they can be treated.

Chapter 7: Development and growth

From the day your baby is born, doctors will be monitoring his weight, length and head size. Growth is a great indicator of overall health, as children who are growing well are usually healthy; on the other hand, poor growth could be a red flag for several health related issues.

How big should my new-born be?

Similar to adults, there's a wide range of different healthy sizes that babies come in. Most new-borns born between thirty eight to forty weeks should weigh somewhere around 5 pounds, 8 ounces or two thousand and five hundred grams and eight pounds, 13 ounces or four thousand grams.

A baby who's lighter or heavier to this average is usually fine, but in some cases they receive extra attention from the hospital staff just to be sure that there are no problems.

Numerous things can impact a baby's size at birth. One of the most critical factors is pregnancy length. Those born close to their due date or even later tend to be bigger in size than those born earlier.

Other factors that influence a baby's size at birth:

Size of parents. It's common for short parents to usually have smaller than average new-borns, while tall parents have larger than average new-borns.

Twins, triplets, etc. Mothers that have had multiple babies at one can count on her babies being smaller than average. This is because their babies had to share their space with their siblings while inside the uterus. Multiples are typically born earlier, which also leads to a smaller than average size at birth.

Birth order. First babies are usually smaller sized than any siblings born later.

Gender. Although the difference at birth isn't as noticeable as in later stages, girls tend to be smaller at birth than boys.

Mother's health. A mother with health issues such as high blood pressure, will usually have a smaller than average sized child at birth. Also, mothers that used cigarettes, alcohol, or other drugs pregnancy can affect negatively their child's weight. Sometimes, weight issues such as obesity can result in babies with higher birth weight. Every condition that can have an impact on the baby's weight and health should be carefully monitored by a doctor. Of course, all mothers should stay away from smoking, alcohol and other illegal drugs while pregnant.

Diet during pregnant. A mother with good nutrition will positively impact his child's health, not only during pregnancy but in later stages too. A less than ideal diet while pregnant can impact how much a baby weighs and how he grows. Gaining weight during pregnancy can increase the chances that the baby will be larger than average.

Baby's health. Medical conditions, including some birth defects and certain infections acquired throughout the pregnancy phase, can all impact a baby's birth weight and growth potential.

Premature babies

Premature babies are usually smaller in size and weight than other babies. A preemie's weight is going to be largely based on how early he was born. Babies are constantly growing while inside the uterus, therefore, any time that he missed means that he has to make up for it in the outside world.

A lot of premature babies are considered to have a "low birth weight" or even "very low birth weight." In medical literature, "low birth weight" means that the child weighs under 5 pounds, 8 ounces (2,500 grams) at birth. This is common for around 1 in every 12 babies born in the United States. When a child is considered as having a "Very low birth weight" it means that he weighs under 3 pounds, 5 ounces (1,500 grams). Most babies with low or really low birth weight are often born prematurely.

Premature babies receive immediate medical attention when they're born, and a pediatric specialist is usually assigned to monitor their health. Many premature babies spend some time in a neonatal intensive care unit while their health is monitored and cared for. Their feeding sometimes requires special attention from the staff as well.

Is it better for babies to be born bigger?

Some time ago, a child born with chubby cheeks and dimpled thighs was considered the standard for a healthy newborn. However, we now know that children born with a larger than average size might need special attention and might even have certain medical conditions.

Some extremely large babies - especially common with overweight or diabetic mothers, might have trouble keeping ideal blood sugar levels for a few days and may need to be fed more often or be administered intravenous glucose to prevent the levels from lowering more.

Is my baby going to lose weight?

Initially, yes. Most babies are born with extra fluid, so it's only natural for them to lose a few ounces when that fluid is dropped after the first days of life. Healthy babies are expected to lose anywhere from 7% to 10% of their birth weight, but are expected to quickly regain that weight around the first 2 weeks.

Throughout their first month, the average new-born will gain around 1 ounce (30 grams) each day and increase 1 to 1½ inches (2.54 to three.81 centimeters) in height. Many new-borns go through an increased growth spurt when they are around 10 days old and then again when they are between 4 and 6 weeks old.

Should I be worried?

New-borns are usually very small, and it can be tough to determine if your baby is gaining weight properly or not. Parents often worry that their baby lose a surprising amount of weight during the first days or if they aren't drinking enough breast of formula milk. If so, you should get in contact with a paediatrician, who may ask you the following:

The amount of feedings per day that your baby gets. Breastfed babies usually eat more than formula-fed babies. It's common for them to feed about 8 or more times during the day while formula babies tend to eat only after 3 to 4 hours. Breastfeeding counsellors can give great suggestions based on the mother's and baby's needs to make feeding sessions more comfortable.

How much your baby is eating. It's typical for new-borns to feed for 10 to 15 minutes, take a few breaks and continue. You should notice that your baby is swallowing and also watch for signs that he's satisfied before ending a feeding session. Monitor closely how many times he's eating throughout the day, as it can be valuable information for paediatricians.

How often your baby pees. On average, a breastfed baby may only need to pee once or twice per day until his mother's milk comes in before the mother's milk is available in. Expect about 6 wet diapers once he starts drinking milk for the first 3 to 5 days. Afterwards, babies typically wet their diapers six to eight times per day.

The number of bowel movements per day. Newborns typically only have one bowel movement per day at first. You'll notice that the poop is dark and tarry at first and then becomes loser and has a green-yellow color after 4-5 days. Babies usually have more bowel movements when breastfed than when formula-fed.

Setting expectations

Being big or small at birth does not always mean that a child is going to be big or small later on in childhood and adulthood. Lots of towering teenagers were born as small premature babies, and the biggest baby in your neighbourhood can end up becoming a petite sized adult.

A better predictor of a baby's eventual height by the time he's an adult, is the size of his parents. Genetics, along with nutrition, play a huge part in determining how a child will grow later in life.

Whether your new-born is born small, large or average, expect him to grow very quickly during the upcoming months.

Conclusion

I hope this book was able to help you gain a better understanding of what to expect from your new-born and his first months so that you can help him transition into a happy and healthy toddler.

Though most parents make lots of mistakes during the many years it takes to raise a child; love, attention, and care will always provide strong support for healthy development.

There is no such thing as "too much information" when it comes to raising a child, so make an effort to learn as much as you can from trusted sources and from people who are already a long way down the road you are traveling now.

Baby Care

A Guide to the Most Important Months of your Baby's Life. Proper Feeding, Sleeping, and Care During the First Year

Copyright 2018 by Joseph R. Parker - All rights reserved.

This document is geared towards providing exact and reliable information in regards to the topic and issue covered. The publication is sold with the idea that the publisher is not required to render accounting, officially permitted, or otherwise, qualified services. If advice is necessary, legal or professional, a practiced individual in the profession should be ordered.

- From a Declaration of Principles which was accepted and approved equally by a Committee of the American Bar Association and a Committee of Publishers and Associations.

In no way is it legal to reproduce, duplicate, or transmit any part of this document in either electronic means or in printed format. Recording of this publication is strictly prohibited and any storage of this document is not allowed unless with written permission from the publisher. All rights reserved.

The information provided herein is stated to be truthful and consistent, in that any liability, in terms of inattention or otherwise, by any usage or abuse of any policies, processes, or directions contained within is the solitary and utter responsibility of the recipient reader. Under no circumstances will any legal responsibility or blame be held against the publisher for any reparation, damages, or monetary loss due to the information herein, either directly or indirectly.

Respective authors own all copyrights not held by the publisher.

The information herein is offered for informational purposes solely, and is universal as so. The presentation of the information is without contract or any type of guarantee assurance.

The trademarks that are used are without any consent, and the publication of the trademark is without permission or backing by the trademark owner. All trademarks and brands within this book are for clarifying purposes only and are the owned by the owners themselves, not affiliated with this document.

Baby Care

A Guide to the Most Important Months of your Baby's Life. Proper Feeding, Sleeping, and Care During the First Year

Copyright 2018 by Joseph R. Parker - All rights reserved.

This document is geared towards providing exact and reliable information in regards to the topic and issue covered. The publication is sold with the idea that the publisher is not required to render accounting, officially permitted, or otherwise, qualified services. If advice is necessary, legal or professional, a practiced individual in the profession should be ordered.

- From a Declaration of Principles which was accepted and approved equally by a Committee of the American Bar Association and a Committee of Publishers and Associations.

In no way is it legal to reproduce, duplicate, or transmit any part of this document in either electronic means or in printed format. Recording of this publication is strictly prohibited and any storage of this document is not allowed unless with written permission from the publisher. All rights reserved.

The information provided herein is stated to be truthful and consistent, in that any liability, in terms of inattention or otherwise, by any usage or abuse of any policies, processes, or directions contained within is the solitary and utter responsibility of the recipient reader. Under no circumstances will any legal responsibility or blame be held against the publisher for any reparation, damages, or monetary loss due to the information herein, either directly or indirectly.

Respective authors own all copyrights not held by the publisher.

The information herein is offered for informational purposes solely, and is universal as so. The presentation of the information is without contract or any type of guarantee assurance.

The trademarks that are used are without any consent, and the publication of the trademark is without permission or backing by the trademark owner. All trademarks and brands within this book are for clarifying purposes only and are the owned by the owners themselves, not affiliated with this document.

Introduction

There's nothing quite like a baby's first months of life, as they are arguably the ones that will have the most impact throughout the first stages of their development: their overall health, mood and energy are all greatly impacted. It's normal for infants to double in weight during the first 5 months of their lives, and by their first year, even their brain size has increased by thirty percent. Who else but a baby is able to grow over 10 inches in a year?

If you're a first-time parent, you're probably starting to feel stressed out about all the things you'd need to do in order to make all of this growth and development happen. The good news for parents is that nature pretty much takes care of things and that it's not necessary to do that much, as the transitions a baby goes through seem to occur almost on schedule. However, there are tougher challenges to face.

There's a lot to your favour: An infant's behavioural patterns are almost hardwired and you can expect your baby's nervous system and responses to be almost 'programmed' to react the way nature intended. The way they cry and how they smile and look at you all tell you things about the way they currently feel, and so, if we learn understand and react accordingly to these, we are almost guaranteed to have an easier time when raising them.

For a long time, neuroscience has been interested in the way that infant's brains work and develop. It's no wonder why, as a baby's brain are extremely plastic. For babies, the challenge lies in how their brain works, since they are 'designed' by nature to behave and react a certain way, in the first year of their lives there is a continuous process of 'rewiring' going on; whether you're trying to teach your baby their first words, or new motor skills, you are helping shape their neural pathways, and they are quick to respond to this new stimuli. In those first months of life, your success as a parent is largely dependent on how you reshape your baby's neural pathways.

If you're afraid that you might be unprepared for the task, especially if you're a new parent, remember that just as babies are 'wired' to react a certain way, so will your parental instincts kick in at the right time, and the more you are well informed about what lies ahead, the quicker it will all click.

Whether you are a first-time parent or a veteran currently waiting for your fourth one, I hope that the advice in this book helps make life a just a bit easier for you and your new family member.

Chapter 1: The first day at home with your baby

You've most likely heard that all baby does is eat, poop, cry, and sleep all day. For a new parent, it might not sound too complicated, but you'll probably be pulling out your hair on more than a couple occasions at first. Being well aware of what you can expect from your baby will make your first days at home together less overwhelming and more enjoyable.

The following advice is aimed primarily at mothers, although dads can also learn some useful things.

Newborn feeding

Since their stomachs are extremely small, newborns tend to eat in small quantities ranging from one to three ounces - frequently. It's usual for most mothers nurse or have a bottle at hand every 2 to 3 hrs; however, some babies are going to be hungry more frequently.

Although it's typical for babies announce their hunger with strong cries, there are some that tend to give subtle cues instead - for example sucking on their fingers, smacking their lips, or turning their heads towards the mother's breast or bottle.

Within their first couple of days, newborns typically lose about seven percent of their bodyweight. Although this is weight loss is completely normal, you will want to feed him every two hrs approximately until he's back at his birth weight.

Newborns are wired to sleep a lot, so you may need to be waking your baby up often so that you can feed. Try and give some gentle encouragement so that he remain awake while eating. If you're having trouble keeping your baby awake, you can try speaking to him, undressing him down to his diapers and rubbing his chest, head or back. The aim is to help you baby get back to birth weight by the time the 2-week check-up arrives.

Baby burps, hiccups, and spit-ups

Some babies need to be burped often, while some burp by themselves and don't need much assistance from you. In case your baby seems to be uncomfortable during or after a feeding session, that's your cue to help him out.

Try burping your child whenever you switch breasts, after feeding two or three ounces, every ten to fifteen minutes of feeding, or whenever your baby's finished eating. After a couple of days of feeding him, you will find a method that works for him.

Avoid banging your baby's back like a drum – doing a gentle circular motion or soft pats will usually be enough. There are many burping positions you can try out, including holding your child with the head resting on your shoulder, sitting him upright in your lap using the fingers of 1 hand supporting the chest and chin area, or putting your baby tummy-down across your lap.

No need to be alarmed by hiccups or spit-ups. Hiccups are common for newborns and do not cause them discomfort. Also, spitting up after and during feedings - in small amounts or what may appear during the entire feeding - is pretty normal.

In case your baby's spitting-up appears excessive or if its followed by him arching his back and/or crying, it could be reflux, which is fairly normal and gets better when your baby develops better head control. However, in some cases where the spitting up seems to be excessive, you might want to consult with a physician, since it might be sigh of gastroesophageal reflux disease (GERD) which usually requires treatment. Whatever's the cause, if your new-born is a "spitter-upper", you might want to keep a few clean cloths nearby.

Baby pee and poop

Expect a breastfed baby to wet diapers at least 4 times every day. If you're feeding your baby a formula, expect them to pee at least 10 times.

Parents often wonder about what a "healthy" number of bowel movements is, but in reality the range can be pretty wide. Breastfed new-borns have a tendency to poop more often than formula-fed ones, since formulas take quite longer to digest. Breastfed babies vary a lot, so don't be surprised if he only poops once every three days or as frequently as once per feeding session. Formula-given babies typically poop a couple of occasions each day, however it can vary in one poop every two days to several times per day. It's important to keep an eye on your new-born's peeing and pooping times, because your physician may ask questions related do this during the first checkup.

The initial bowel motions - usually occurring during the very first day or more, frequently while you still haven't left the hospital - are known as meconium. These first poops possess a black, almost tar-like consistency. Those that follow will not look similar to grown-up poop either, so do not be surprised and be ready for green, light brown, or mustard-yellow poops from your breastfed newborn. Formula fed baby poop is commonly pastier and varies in colour. Call your physician if you notice that your baby's stool contains whitish mucus or streaks or flecks of red, which could indicate an issue. (Red is an indication of bloodstream in poop.)

Normal poop consistency also varies from very soft to watery, with breastfed babies usually having looser stools. This may be easily mistaken for diarrhea. The important thing is to keep an eye out for anything that's a change from your newborn's typical poops– which can be tricky whenever your baby is first developing a pattern.

If you are feeling confused, keep in mind this: when talking about pooping, eating, sleeping habits, or crying, the normal range is quite wide and what's most important to consider are sudden changes - and that is when you should consult with a pediatrician.

Crying

There is no avoiding this one: Your newborn will cry often. How frequently, how hard, and how long it will last varies and tends to change over time.

For the first couple of days, many newborns are remarkably quiet and sleepy. But by the time they are 2 or 3 weeks old, the average newborn will cry for two hrs each day. (Crying frequency and duration typically increases until they reach eight weeks of age and then diminishes steadily.)

With time, it'll get simpler to determine why your child is crying. At the first stages, it's a good idea to go through common culprits such as wet or soiled diapers, hunger or tiredness, and you'll most likely find the cause. In some cases, a common reason for excessive crying can be overstimulation. Some babies get picky when they are dealing with an excessive amount of commotion or activity.

You will see that in certain occasions, however, whenever your baby cries without any obvious cause, and you will need to find out what soothes him. Remember: there's no such thing as 'spoiling your child' at these very early stage, so react to the cries with proper attention and affection.

If you're having a hard time finding out why your baby is crying and you start to feel helpless, frustrated, or incompetent, try to take it easy on yourself. Every parent, even veteran ones, have been there at some point. Sure, there will be times when your baby's needs are easy to understand, but often you'll find be left wondering about what's going on!

Newborn sleep

Your baby's small tummy will probably keep him from sleeping for more than a couple of hrs at any given time before he wakes up and asks for something to eat. All of those short naps your baby is taking will add up, and your newborn will typically sleep around 18 hrs every day. You might want to track where and when your child sleeps, to recognize patterns and answer any questions your physician might make.

Fortunately, newborns possess the amazing ability to go to sleep virtually anywhere - within the vehicle seat, baby carrier, bassinet, and even in your arms. Many babies like the snug fit of the vehicle seat or baby carrier for sleeping, since the close confines help remind them of the womb. This is exactly why a lot of newborns love being swaddled, too. By snuggly wrapping them up, you are mimicking the atmosphere your child has been used to, and prevents reflexive jerks from his limbs from waking him up.

Regardless of when or where your child sleeps, always remember to lay him on his back and take away all loose blankets, as well as pillows, quilts, and toys. This is mainly a preventive measure for Sudden Infant Death Syndrome (SIDS). Also, avoid leaving a snoozing baby unwatched on the couch or bed as the chances of him moving and falling are always present, even when your infant isn't able to roll on his own yet.

When your baby is asleep, expect to hear strange noises from him. Although it could sound like your child has a cold, it may actually be due to the fact that they naturally breathe from the nose and there's a bit of blockage due to mucus build-up. Since he can't clean his nasal passages on his own yet, you can use a bulb syringe to clear out any blockage.

Baby breathing

Another habit you'll notice in your baby is periodic breathing. Your child may breathe rapidly, pause for a moment (usually a few seconds), then start breathing again. Although completely normal, some parents that aren't that aren't aware of periodic breathing might get very worried.

However, the following signs aren't normal and warrant contacting your baby's physician as soon as possible:

-Grunting

-Nostrils flaring

-Retractions at the chest area.

-Consistently fast breathing

-Wheezing coming from her chest (instead of her nose or throat, which is a common flag of congestion)

-Heavy, noisy breathing (audible wheezes, whizzing sounds, or crackly sounds during the inhalation and exhalation process)

-Pauses that are longer than ten to fifteen seconds between breaths.

Bathing

Keeping the baby clean within the first few days is fairly simple. For the time being, you will not need to use the baby bathtub. If your baby's umbilical cord stump continues to be hanging on, avoid immersing it in water. Sponge baths will suffice to help keep a baby clean for those first weeks. Keep in mind that an excessive amount of bathing can be counterproductive as it can have negative side effects such as drying up your baby's skin.

It's recommended to use a warm and damp cloth or unscented baby wipes to lightly wipe around areas where breast milk, formula or moisture tends to accumulate without you noticing, such as neck folds and the genital area. If you see any redness or irritation within the diaper area, a bit of diaper cream or petroleum jelly can help.

Don't expect your new-born baby's skin to look just like the baby skin in the commercials, since many newborns usually have several minor skin irritations, with newborn rash, cradle cap, peeling, or general dryness being the most common. This is expected for anyone that has just recently emerged from a nine-month bath in amniotic fluid! You may also notice some hair in unexpected places such as the back and shoulders – which usually falls out after a few days or weeks.

Newborn clothes

Cute or funny outfits will have to take a back seat to comfort and ease in the first weeks. Prioritize clothes that are simple to change, and work great for your baby's many naps. A lot of parents use a mixture of shirts, single piece bodysuits, and footed pajamas, along with a sleep sack when there's cold temperature or during the night.

You might find that your new-born dislikes getting clothes pulled over his head. If you notice that your baby cries after each clothe change, it might be due to umbilical cord stump sensitivity. In those cases, one-piece outfits that snap easily at the sides can be helpful. For warmth, a lot of hospitals send newborn babies home with hats, but this is not necessary unless temperatures are low.

Make use of your instincts: we all have an internal thermostat that can help us gauge the number of layers to use. Lots of people stick to the classic advice of - "whatever you are wearing plus one" for babies. While in doubt, you can use a blanket or hat – which are easy to take off in case your baby feels warm.

Newborn gear

During the pregnancy months, most parents probably have accumulated a little mountain of baby gear. For the time being, you won't be using most of it. The most important things you'll need is a safe place for your newborn to sleep and a secure car seat for the ride home. Extra stuff, for example bouncy seats, activity mats, toys, along with other baby gear will be useful at some point, but try not to be worried about them now. The baby's needs at this time are all basic and not complex.

The transition home

The first time you bring a baby home makes for a life-altering change, and parents should not expect to be prepared as soon they walk-through the doorway. It can actually take anywhere from a few weeks to several months for parents to feel at ease. While you are navigating through this adjustment phase, make sure that you're going easy on yourself and pay little attention to opinions from others about how exactly things should or shouldn't be.

If you're a mother, your body is still coping with fluctuating hormonal levels, healing from having a baby, and you may be seriously sleep-deprived. Also, your mind is still getting used to this new stage of your life. You might laugh, cry, be frustrated, get excited, and feel an array of feelings within a small timeframe. You will most likely discover that taking care of a baby - simple as his needs may be – take up a lot of your time, which can make it hard to pay attention to your own most basic ones.

The vast majority of new moms experience what's called "baby blues" throughout the hormonal ride occur the first days after giving birth. Fortunately, baby blues tend to fade away quickly, sometimes within two or three days. All new mothers should be aware of them, though, as well as any signs of postpartum depression (PPD).

When compared to baby blues, postpartum depression lasts longer and can be a more serious condition. PPD affects around 10 % women. Seeking out professional help and getting treatment is very important for you, your partner and your new baby.

One effective method to combat baby blues is to make sure to leave small bits of time for yourself. You can enlist the help of your partner, family members, or friends to handle chores and errands. Don't be shy when asking them to help with basic things such as doing groceries, bring meals, or doing the laundry

While your new-born sleeps, feel free to use that time to rest, shower or watch your favourite TV show. Anything that helps you can recharge your batteries between all those diaper changes and feeding.

Changes to expect in your body

After giving birth, your body will go through huge physical changes. In the first 72 hrs you will start producing milk. Frequently, this coincides with your first days back home. So far you have been producing the coveted colostrum, which is the first milk that your body produces during pregnancy, which is yellower than breast milk. What colostrum lacks in volume, it makes up in power, since it's full of antibodies and acts as your baby's first vaccination.

When your breasts become noticeably larger, firmer, and heavier, you'll know that you'll begin producing real milk. This is where engorgement typically occurs.

Even though most people assume that breastfeeding starts naturally, it isn't rare for there to be a few issues in the road - especially in early stages. Even mothers that were coached by a lactation consultant or nurse in the hospital might need more help once they're home. With some practice, you'll start learning the finer points - from getting your baby to latch perfectly to identifying the best hold for both of you.

Many mothers complain that breastfeeding makes their nipples really sore. Try out a few different positions to avoid aching and cracking. Washing your breasts with water, applying pure lanolin cream after breastfeeding (it's not necessary to remove the cream before feeding), using a few drops of breast milk like nipple moisturizer, or icing your breasts might help alleviate the soreness.

If you are unsure whether your newborn is hungry or not, focus on whether he really swallows or not whenever he's sucking on your breast. In many cases, babies like to suck on their mother's breast for self-soothing purposes instead of nursing. There's no harm in offering her own thumb for comfort so that your nipples can take a break.

If you have made the decision not to breastfeed, get advice from your physician or better yet, a lactation consultant if you can find one near your area, about the easiest method to suppress lactation. Once the milk starts coming in, a lot of mothers are surprised to find that it may be difficult to shut down production without discomfort.

Mothers that stop lactating typically experience engorgement discomfort. It's normal for the discomfort to peak about 3 to 5 days after childbirth and then decrease. To handle the temporary discomfort, you can try using over-the-counter pain relievers, ice packs, along with special supportive bras. A decongestant can also be helpful as it speeds up the process by drying out body tissues.

You'll most likely be sore if you had a regular vaginal delivery. In case there was any tearing or an episiotomy, it might even be extra painful. You can apply a cloth-covered ice pack to help combat the swelling. Some women have great success using witch hazel pads to reduce the inflammation.

When going to the bathroom, basic things such as wiping may be painful. You can try using a squirt water bottle instead. A lot of women experience severe constipation after delivery, so a diet rich in fibre can help. Also, for around six days after delivery you'll most likely need to use a sanitary napkin to soak up the normal bleeding and discharge (also known as lochia).

In case that you had a c-section, which is considered a major abdominal surgery, you'll need assistance with almost everything for 1-3 weeks. You will probably find it very hard to do basic household tasks and even feed your baby or change diapers. Many doctors recommend avoiding lifting anything heavier than an average size new-born baby until the first postpartum check-up.

You'll most likely leave the hospital with some type medication to alleviate the pain, and it's important to keep track of which one you're taking and when. Avoid trying to feel brave, and avoid taking the medication;

you might be in such discomfort that even simple interaction with your baby becomes difficult.

Call your physician if you see bloodstream or pus seeping from the surgery area, as that may be a strong sign of an infection or clot. Similar as if had a vaginal delivery, you will want to avoid straining on the toilet, and you may want to use stool softener and eat a fibre rich diet.

For first time mothers, probably the most shocking reasons about their post pregnancy bodies might be the fact that they could still look pregnant. If that's the case, do not worry, as it often takes days - or several weeks - for your skin (especially at the belly area) to completely recover. Meanwhile, it's perfectly normal to continue using maternity clothes after delivery.

Taking your baby out of home

A lot of parents are worried about taking their babies outside for the first time after they arrive home from the hospital. There are some cultures that have the tradition of making moms and babies stay at home for the first month or longer. However, in reality there isn't any medical reason to not take your young baby outside. Being outside can be a great change of pace for both parents and their babies. The tricky part is avoiding exposure to others, as this is what may cause them to become sick.

To prevent exposing your child to harmful germs, limit time spent in close quarters with crowds. Make certain that anybody who would like to hold or touch your child washes his hands. Finally, avoid anybody who's sick. Don't be afraid to ask people that want to hold your child if they've washed their hands or if they've been sick recently.

As your baby grows, he'll probably be extremely keen on anything outside your home, and will be amazed at the new views, sounds, and smells. A great time to go outside is whenever your baby is feeling happy, as they will get out more of the experience. If you plan on going outside, a good time can also be after feeding and changing diapers as the probably will be in a good mood and will be able to relax.

If you are planning on taking your baby outside for over an hour, it would be best to be well prepared and stock your baby bag with fresh clothes, and eating/cleaning supplies.

Dress your child appropriately if you are spending some time outdoors. If it is chilly, be sure to cover well the head, feet and hands. On the other hand, if it's a bit hot and sunny outside, make sure that you safeguard your baby well by using sunscreen and light garments.

Always be careful with temperature extremes. Depending on your baby's age and the climate outside, 20 degrees is usually too cold and 90 degrees might be hot for him to tolerate.

Chapter 2: All about baby sleep

Babies sleep a great deal – and their sleeping schedules might unexpectedly change from one week to the next, depending on where they are at in their development. The end result? Plenty of sleep for the baby along with a very irregular - and tiring - agenda for you. You'll most likely be up several occasions throughout the night to alter, feed, and soothe him.

Why baby sleep patterns are unpredictable

Baby sleep cycles are far shorter than individuals of adults, and they spend a lot of time in the Rapid Eye Moment (REM) phase of sleep, which is considered essential to the incredibly fast development happening in their brains.

All of this unpredictability in their sleeping patterns is an important phase for the baby that fortunately doesn't last long in the majority of cases - although to your sleep-deprived mind it might seem like an eternity!

When will my baby start sleeping for longer periods of time?

Once they reach six to eight weeks of age, most babies start to sleep for shorter periods throughout the day and for longer ones during the night, though most will keep waking up and ask to be fed at night. At this point, they will be having shorter periods of REM sleep, and will spend a longer time in deep, non-REM sleep.

Most experts mention that between the first 4 and 6 months, most babies are able to handle sleeping for eight to twelve hours during the night. If you're lucky, your baby might start sleeping for longer without waking up during the night as early as 6 weeks, but on average, most babies don't reach this milestone until they are at least five to six months old, and a few still get up during the night for a few more months. The good news for parents is that they can assist their child to reach the milestone sooner, by teaching a few simple sleeping habits from the beginning.

Establishing good baby sleep habits

Here's some practical advice to help your baby develop great sleeping habits:

Let your baby take frequent naps. For those initial 6 to 8 weeks, most babies will have a hard time staying awake for more than a couple of hours at a time. Should you wait more than that to help your baby fall asleep, he may start developing sleeping issues. To avoid this, make sure that your baby is taking frequent naps during the day.

Teaching the difference between night and day. For some unfortunate parents, their babies can be night owls (something that mothers might be aware of during the pregnancy months) and will be wide awake while they're only thinking about get some shut-eye. The first days with your newborn baby, there's not much that you can do about this, but after 2-3 weeks have gone by, you can help him distinguish between night and day.

When your baby is alert and awake throughout the day, interact and have fun with him whenever you can, keep your house (and the baby's room) well lit, and forget about minimizing regular daytime noises such as the phone, music, or dishwasher. If your baby has a tendency to sleep while feeding, wake him up.

At night time, avoid playing with your baby when he wakes up. Avoid bright lights around the house and keep the noise level low, and don't talk to him too much when preparing him for sleep. It won't be long for his body to figure out that night time is perfect for sleeping.

Identifying signs that your baby is tired. Keep an eye out for any signs that your baby wants to go to sleep: is he rubbing his eyes, pulling on his ears, or acting a bit moody? All of these are good indicators of sleepiness, and whenever you notice any of them, avoid delaying putting him to sleep. You will soon create a sixth sense regarding your baby's daily rhythms and patterns, and you will know instinctively when he's ready to take a good nap.

Sleeping routines for your baby. It's never too late to develop a healthy bed time routine for your baby. There are simple things you can do to help him understand that sleep time is approaching. Some ideas can be singing a lullaby while getting him changed for bed, and giving a goodnight kiss and hug.

Teach your baby to go to sleep by himself. When he's six to eight days weeks old, don't be afraid to give your baby the opportunity to learn how to go sleep by himself. Many parents try rocking or nursing their babies to sleep as it tends to work and make them fall asleep quickly. Unfortunately, this does nothing to help your baby learn how to sleep by himself, and might prove to be counterproductive as it will be difficult for him to shake off this habit later on. If you're always rocking your baby to sleep, why would he expect anything different when he's 5 or 6 months old?

This strategy is a bit controversial among parents because some believe that rocking or nursing their babies to sleep is a harmless method, but in reality it acts only as a short-term solution and you might find yourself getting up several times during the night to rock your baby just so he can go to sleep again.

When do babies start sleeping through the night?

Some parents start getting worried that their babies aren't sleeping through the night once they're 6 months old. If you're baby now sleeps for eight or more hrs during the night, this means he's found out a way how to get back to sleep by himself - an indication that you are raising a great sleeper. Congratulations!

In case your baby is not yet sleeping for eight straight hrs. or more during the night, you are definitively not alone on this. A lot of babies still wake during the night, usually asking to be fed during the night at the 6- to 9- month stage.

Babies at this stage don't always wake up because they are hungry. Even adults tend to wake up several times every night, but we are able to put ourselves back to sleep every time, so quickly, in fact, that we rarely remember in the morning. In case your baby has not mastered this skill yet, he'll wake up several times during the night and cry even if he isn't hungry.

When is my baby ready for sleep training?

If your baby is at the 5-6 month stage and he has not yet settled right into a sleep pattern that matches your own, now may well be a great time teach him some form of sleep training. Sleep training techniques might help your child fall asleep easier and sleep for extended periods during the night.

Here's three of the most effective sleep training methods:

They 'cry out' strategy

Advocates of this sleep training technique mention that it's okay for your baby to cry whenever you put him to sleep, even though they don't advocate letting an infant cry indefinitely. Typically, these techniques suggest putting your child to sleep when he's still awake and allowing short periods of crying interspersed with comforting (but avoiding picking up) your baby.

The 'no tears' strategy

Sleep training advocates of this method encourage a far more gradual approach - soothing the infant to sleep and offering comfort only once he starts crying. After a while, you can back off on the time you take to comfort him.

The 'fading' strategy

Fading, also referred to as adult fading, falls right in the middle of the spectrum among the typical sleep training techniques. In fading, parents progressively diminish their bed time role to by keeping close to their baby until he falls asleep and progressively away from the crib every night. Another way of using fading is to check on your child and reassure him (without holding him) every 5-10 minutes until he falls asleep. The aim is to give him enough time so that he learns how to soothe himself.

If you're wondering which technique to try, it really depends on which strategy works with your parenting philosophy or lifestyle and whatever your baby will respond the best to. Try them out and observe carefully how your baby reacts. Sleep training techniques have been continuously debated by researchers, and while there is not a definite answer on which is the best method, they all agree that consistency appears to be key. Whichever sleep training method you find that your baby responds great to, try and follow through on with it.

Why your child might have problems remaining asleep

Many babies at around 6 to 12 month mark suddenly start having difficulties when falling asleep. This may happen to your baby even if he was a great sleeper before. Why? Sleep disturbances are frequently related to reaching major milestones in cognitive and motor development and with separation anxiety as well.

When your child reaches 6 to 9 months of age, he might start to learn how to sit up, crawl, or even walk in some cases. Unsurprisingly, he might feel that he'd like to practice his new skills at night time and could get so excited to try again that he'll wake up just to see if he can practice a bit more.

Stress and anxiety could also be causing sleeping issues. If your baby hasn't been properly sleep trained, he'll feel distressed upon waking up and finding out that his parents aren't nearby.

Finally, the discomfort caused by teething may be waking him up.

While it can be hard to determine exactly what's causing your child to wake up, always keep in mind that there are plenty of good reasons at this stage. So it is best to adjust your expectations and be a little flexible.

Keep in mind that each child differs. Some of them will have a much easier time sleeping than others. And you will need to adapt with the changes whenever travel, illness, and important events clash with sleep patterns.

If your child has reached 6 to 9 months of age and is having trouble going to sleep, you can try the following:

Keep your baby on a consistent schedule. You'll both take advantage of using a regular sleeping schedule which includes set occasions for both bed and naps. That does not mean your child needs to eat his last meal at exactly 7:15 every single day, but try and do your best to stick to a predictable schedule that works for your lifestyle. In case your baby naps, eats, plays, and gets ready for bed at similar times every single day, he'll be more likely to go to sleep easily.

Remove any distractions at night. Take away anything that's remotely eye catching that's nearby your baby's crib at night. Just like adults, babies sleep best in rooms that are completely dark. If there's any house or street sounds, consider using a fan or white noise machine to muffle them out. Turn off all screens in the bedroom, including TVs and even small mobile devices.

Try putting him to sleep earlier. In case your baby's accustomed to sleeping after 8:30 p.m. and has a hard time winding down before that, try gradually putting him to sleep a few minutes earlier. Start with 20 minutes and do 10 minute increments with each successful day.

Baby and small child sleep timeline

This timeline will give you a good idea of how much sleep children typically need from their first days of life up to their third year and how sleep and nap patterns change as they develop.

Newborns. Usually sleep for about 17 hrs within a 24-hour period. There is no predictable pattern for your new-born's sleep, and he'll probably sleep anywhere from a few mins to a few hours at any given time. The main reason for waking up at this stage is to refill his little tummy.

1 month. The average is still around 17 hrs. This is when babies start to determine the main differences between night and day. By now he's probably doing most of his shut-eye during the night time hrs but nonetheless he'll probably be sleeping a great deal throughout the day.

2 months. Around 16 to 17 hrs. Though more alert and social, most babies this age still take 3 to 4 (or maybe more) naps each day. Your child may begin skipping one feeding session at night time at this point.

3 months. Around 16 hrs. Some, but, not every baby at this stage can sleep for lengthy stretches of 6 to 8 hrs during the night. Most need to take around three daytime naps.

6 months. Around 15 hrs. During the night, babies typically log around 9-10 hrs of sleep. Daytime naps might now lower to 2 or 1 in the morning and another in the afternoon (although it's not uncommon for some babies to take three or even four short naps).

9-10 months. Around 14 to fifteen hrs, with an average of 11 of those being at night-time. 70 to 80 % of babies this age are actually sleeping without waking up during the night (which would usually be from 8-12 hours straight). Your child is most likely still taking two solid naps each day, at the morning and mid-day. At this point, he might have difficulties going to sleep and remaining asleep due to separation anxiety.

12 months. Around 14 hrs. One-year-olds frequently sleep for around 11 hrs during the night, plus two daytime naps (which might become shorter and shorter).

18 months. Around 13 to 14 hrs. At this point, your child's morning nap is most likely history. However, he's prone to hold on to the mid-day nap for a few years. Most children this age still sleep for about 11 hrs. during the night.

2 years. Around 11 to 14 hrs. Most 2-year-olds still take their afternoon naps and sleep around ten to twelve hrs at night-time. Your little rebel may resist sleeping now and, if he's no longer using a crib, may get out of bed after tucking him in.

3 years. Around 10 to 13 hrs. Your pre-schooler can always take a mid-day nap, however, many kids this age drop naps altogether. Frequently they compensate this by snoozing longer during the night. Many have switched from the crib to a regular kid sized bed at this point.

Chapter 3: Dealing with separation anxiety

There's no way around the fact that your baby will experience separation anxiety to a degree at some point. This is actually a normal stage of their emotional development that starts when babies start to realize that their parents and things exist even if they are not present – a concept known as "object permanence."

At the early stages, most babies or toddlers can show signs of having real anxiety and will show discomfort at the suspicion or reality of being separated from their parents. Separation anxiety has a very strong purpose in evolutionary terms, and it makes sense: a baby, being defenseless, would naturally get upset over being taken away from the person that protects him and keeps him from harm.

In lots of ways, attitudes about babies and separations are largely cultural. Western countries have a tendency to stress autonomy from a very young age. However in a number of other cultures, infants are hardly ever separated from their mothers during their first year of life.

Whatever the culture, there's no denying that separation anxiety can be very frustrating for babies and their parents. The good thing is that this type of anxiety is temporal - and you can do certain things to make it more manageable without impacting negatively your child's development. Meanwhile, take a moment to appreciate that at this point in time you're the most important thing in the world for your baby.

At what point does it occur?

Babies can display indicators of separation anxiety as soon as six or seven months of age, and on average it peaks at around 10 to 18 months, and will greatly diminish by the time they reach their second birthday.

Generally, this type of anxiety often strikes whenever you leave your infant when going to work or to run errands.

Your child may also experience stress and anxiety during the night, when he's securely tucked in his crib while you're in the room next to him. The discomfort usually eases when infants reach 2 years of age.

How can parents help?

There are many steps you can take to assist your child through stress and anxiety:

Arrange childcare with individuals familiar to your child. If you need to leave your child - whenever you go back to work, for instance - try having people he already knows, like his aunt or a grandparent take care of him. Your baby will still experience a degree of separation anxiety, as there's nothing quite like being close to his parents, but it can help a lot nonetheless. Your child can always protest, but he may adapt to your absence easier when encircled by well-known faces.

Get him to know new caregivers. Sometimes, there will be no familiar faces to take care of your child in your absence. The best thing you can do whenever you need to leave your child with someone he doesn't know is to provide him with an opportunity to become familiar with the new caregiver while you are still around.

Have a goodbye routine. You can prepare a short and sweet routine that you can do every time you say goodbye to your baby. The predictability of the routine will help him build trust in his own ability when being separated from you and performing the same action will make him know what to expect without being caught by surprise.

Preparing your baby for separations

Just like with any other transition, it's better to take a gradual approach. Whether you need to leave your baby with a relative or a paid caretaker, try these suggestions:

Practicing at home first. It will likely be easier for your child to handle your absence if he's the one that initiates the separation first. Allow him to crawl off and away to another room by herself (one where you are sure he'll be secure without supervision briefly), and wait a few minutes before going near him again.

Provide your baby with enough time to get comfortable. If you're going to hire a baby sitter, try and have her visit your house to meet and play with your baby for a few times before you leave them alone without you nearby. The first time you need to be leave your baby with her, ask the sitter to arrive earlier – 30 mins will do. This will ensure that she and your baby will be well engaged before you leave home. You can use a similar approach if you're leaving your baby with a friend or relative – just make sure to arrive earlier so that he feels comfortable with them thanks to your presence.

Always remember to say goodbye. Make sure to make it a habit to kiss, hug, and talk to your child before leaving. Just a few key things: avoid holding him and do not prolong your goodbyes. Many parents like to sneak out the house so that the baby doesn't notice their departure. This can be counterproductive as your baby will think you simply disappeared out of his life.

No turning back. Returning after saying goodbye just to give one more kiss or hug or repeated into the daycare center to check how your child is doing will only make it harder for everyone involved, including the caregiver.

Consider using a trial period. Limit the first time you are separated from your baby to an hour or two. As both you and your baby become acquainted with the sitter or whomever is taking care of him, you can continue to extend the time.

Dealing with your child's clinginess

Separation anxiety is tough on both babies and their parents, and can cause lots of stress if the child is really having a tough time when they leave or appears to have a preference for one parent over the other. Lots of parents feel guilty about leaving their children with someone that's not them or their partner and are constantly worried about them while they're away. If you find that your child wants your attention constantly, you might feel exhausted, annoyed, and even resentful at times.

These feelings are normal. Keep reminding yourself that the separation anxiety phase is temporary: at this stage your baby is learning how to trust you and at the same time is developing important independence skills. An interesting thing remember for all parents that might be feeling overwhelmed is that separation anxiety is actually positive - a sign of healthy attachment and a good relationship between you and your baby.

Chapter 4: How to properly feed your baby

Parents, especially first timers, wonder all the time if they are feeding their babies properly or not. There are lots of questions about what is best for their healthy development, the pros and cons of breast milk vs formulas, when to introduce solids, etc.

To start off let's take a look at the timeline below so that you have a general idea of what works best at each stage of your baby's first year. Remember that each child is different and there is no way to know accurately how their bodies will respond to food. It's recommended to consult with your paediatrician before making starting a diet plan for your baby or making any major changes.

0 to 4 Months

What to feed your baby: Breast milk or Formula only.

In the first 4 months of their lives, babies haven't got a fully functional digestive system yet. They can't digest any solid foods at this point. Nature has provided babies with an extrusion reflex which stops them from digesting any solids. They also have a rooting reflex that helps them find their mother's breast.

Breastfed babies: If you're breastfeeding your baby then it is advisable to provide him with all the milk they need. It is possible to assess whether your child has had enough milk or not. For example, following a feeding session, your breast will feel soft and the baby will seem to be very relaxed. Over time, the baby's weight can be a great assessing factor too because he should consistently put on weight if he's getting enough milk. Furthermore, the amount of stools he passes every day is another way of figuring out whether he's getting enough nourishment or not.

Formula fed babies: Since formulas tend to be less nourishing than their mother's milk, babies usually demand more feeding sessions. So, be ready to feed your child on multiple occasions throughout the day. However, the diet plan of babies on formula milk can alter pretty rapidly. A good rule of thumb is to offer your baby 2.5 ounces of formula per pound of bodyweight and not to give your baby more than 32 ounces per day.

At this stage it's important to stay away from solids unless your paediatrician says otherwise.

4 to 6 months

What to feed your baby: Continue using the breast milk or formula. Soft cereals can be introduced.

At this stage, there are several developmental milestones that will let you know if your baby is able to eat solids. Some of these are: losing the extrusion reflex, being able to sit with some support, the ability to hold his neck steady, and the ability to move his head back and forth. If you notice these signs, don't delay: When your child reaches 5-6 months of age, his body's iron stores will begin to run out, and he will require more than what he's been getting from formulas or breast milk.

Pediatricians recommend introducing grain cereal first, since it's the grain least prone to cause allergic reactions. You can start by blending a teaspoon of cereal with several tablespoons of breast milk or formula, and feeding your child using a spoon. At first, he'll probably have just a bite or two. You can work your way towards using more cereal, and feeding it to your baby 2 to 3 times/day. Avoid introducing cereal that contains barley, wheat, or oatmeal until he reaches 6 months. You should continue nursing or bottle-feeding -- cereal should only be a supplement to the milk at this time, not a replacement.

Every time you introduce a new food, wait a minimum of 72 hours if you would like to introduce another one. Your baby may have hypersensitive reactions to certain foods, and introducing them this way can make it much easier to determine which ones he's reacting adversely to.

6 to 8 months

What to feed your baby: Breast or formula milk. Soft cereals, pureed vegetables/fruits and some juices.

When your child reaches his sixth month of age, you should begin to introduce vegetables and fruit. Because infants possess a natural preference for sweet foods, many pediatricians suggest presenting veggies first-- otherwise, your child might keep asking for bananas and won't give carrots an opportunity.

Since yellow and orange vegetables are sweeter than eco-friendly ones, carrots, yams, and butternut squash tend to be the best vegetables to introduce first. If your baby spits out her first mouthful of green spinach, keep trying: consistent exposure can convert the most stubborn baby. Begin with strained or pureed vegetables and then introduced mashed ones. Servings should progressively increase from a couple of teaspoons only to approximately two tablespoons, two times per day.

After your baby has sampled a number of vegetables, you can introduce fruit. (Begin small and build up to 2 tablespoons, twice per day.) Stay away from using sweetened treats like cobblers and puddings - the additional fat and sugar add empty calories and may cause your baby to avoid fruits.

Juice is okay occasionally, but it shouldn't be used as a replacement for the fruit itself as it lacks fiber along with other nutrients, and the concentrated sugars can spoil a child and make him prefer it to breast milk or formula – which is still the most essential component of his diet. The American Academy of Pediatrics suggests serving a maximum of four ounces of juice each day, diluted half and half with water if you are offering it frequently. Citrus juice at this point is way too acidic for many babies, and a few other juices such as apple and pear juice can be hard to digest. Research conducted recently has found that white-colored grape juice is the least prone to cause diarrhea and cramping.

7 to 10 months

What to feed your baby: Breast or formula milk. Cereals, tiny pieces of vegetables/fruits, juices, and sometimes cheese and eggs.

Before reaching this stage, your child has been happy eating mushy stuff. But that may change soon, and don't be surprised if he starts eyeing out your dinner plate – he's probably ready for the next feeding stage. It's very important to expose your baby to lumpy foods, as they may develop an oral aversion to such textures if they haven't by the time they reach their twelfth month. Their gag reflex will kick in when they try out foods with unfamiliar textures.

Solid choices for their first lumpy foods can be toast strips, well-cooked pasta, tiny bits of fruit, and well-cooked chopped vegetables. Exercise caution: Several foods, for example nuts, raisins, grapes, and hotdogs, present a choking hazard for children under five years.

By the eight month, breast milk or formula should continue to constitute a large part of your child's diet (3 to 5 breast-feedings or 24 to 32 ounces of formula/day). At this time, however, your baby requires additional protein sources and more iron. Meat can offer both--but your baby might not enjoy it on the first tasting. If you wish to introduce meat, try mixing just a little of it pureed together with her favourite vegetable, and try to build up to two tablespoons each day. Instead of meat you could try using pureed brans, as they are full of nutrients and easy for your baby to enjoy.

10 to 12 months

What to feed your baby: Breast or formula milk. Cereals, cubed vegetables/fruits and some juices, meat, cheese, eggs and yogurt.

As the baby gets closer to his twelfth month, his attitude regarding diet habits will change too. For example, he'll insist on feeding himself. To make things simpler, serve thick-textured foods such as mashed potatoes and casseroles, all of which that are easy to eat with a spoon. If you haven't before, it can be a great time to introduce meat, chicken, or fish.

At 12 months of age, your baby can drink breast milk, whole milk, or enriched soy milk from the cup. (Avoid Low-fat milk until he's 2 years old) By now, his diet is going to be almost as varied as your own: six servings of grains, 2 to 3 of cubed fruits, 2 to 3 of vegetables, and up to three glasses of milk.

At this point your child has mastered the basic food groups, and you can start promoting healthy diet habits. Setting an example yourself works more effectively than pushing him to swallow every bite of strained vegetables. Eat well, eat together, and focus on making mealtime a relaxed, enjoyable time for everyone at the table.

Breastfeeding basics

Those breastfeeding moms make it look so easy that it can make you feel a bit jealous! Without skipping a beat of their conversation or while grabbing a bite of their lunch, they just open a button and latch the baby perfectly. At first, it could take a number of tries to get your baby in to the right position - but keep trying. It's vital to know how to get a good latch, since improper latching is by far the number one cause for breast discomfort. Your baby's mouth should fully cover your nipple and also the areola, to ensure that the baby's mouth, tongue and lips massage milk from your milk glands. (Sucking the nipple only will leave your infant hungry since the glands that secrete the milk will not be properly compressed. It will probably make your nipples sore and cracked too.)

Here's a few ways to perfect the latch:

Hold your child facing your breasts, and place the front of his body facing yours, tummy to tummy. Make sure that the head is properly in line with the rest of his body to make swallowing easier.

Tickle your baby's lip together with your nipple to encourage him to open his mouth very wide, similar to a yawn. In case your baby isn't opening his mouth, try putting some milk on his lips.

If your baby is turning away, you can try and use his rooting reflex to your advantage by stroking the cheek on the side nearest to you. This often makes babies turn their heads towards your breast.

If your baby's mouth is wide open, you can bring them close towards your breast. Don't lean over and push your breast into baby's mouth – have your baby make a bit of effort. Keep your hands on your breast until your baby is grasping it and sucking correctly.

You'll know that your baby has latched properly when his chin and nosetip are touching your breast. His lips should be flared outwards (think fish lips), instead of tucked in. Make sure that your child isn't sucking on his lower lip or tongue by pulling the lower lip down.

Positions for Breastfeeding

Here's some of the most popular and efficient positions for breastfeeding. Due to the nature of audiobooks, we recommend doing a quick search online to get a visual aid and be able to replicate these with more precision.

Side-lying: this is a great position for night-time feeding sessions. Start by lying on your side with a pillow under your head for support. Your child should be facing you, with his head in line with the nipple. With your free hand, cup your breast if necessary. To hold your baby closer, you can try putting a small pillow behind his back.

Cradle hold: place your child in a way that his head is resting in your elbow's bend, on the arm of the side you'll be using for breastfeeding. Use the same hand to support the rest of his body. You can then use the other hand to compress your breast gently so that its nipple points towards the baby.

Football hold: your child's legs should be carefully tucked under your arm that's on the same side as the breast you're using. Hold your child with that arm (you can use a pillow to help lift your baby) and cup your breast with your other hand.

Breastfeeding sessions

While you might have heard that short feeding sessions helps avoid soreness and cracking, that's usually caused by using a suboptimal position. So rather than setting a time limit on every feed, let your baby take his time (and expect the first feedings to be a bit on the longer side).

On average, sessions typically last twenty to thirty minutes. But bear in mind, that's just a rough estimate. Your child might take much more time in the first weeks and during growth spurts.

Drain one breast fully. Ideally, one breast should be completely drained after each feeding session. This is more important than making your baby feed on both breasts. This is because hind milk – which is the milk that comes at the end – tends to be full of nutrients and healthy fats. So don't pull the plug early. Rather, wait until your child seems to be ready to quit on the first breast, then offer (but don't pressure) breast two. If baby drains one breast and doesn't want anymore, start the next feeding session with the other breast.

Watch for signs that your baby is done. Finish the feeding session when the baby let's go of your nipple. In case he doesn't, divert your attention to his "suck-swallow pattern". If you notice that it slows down to four sucks per swallow, that's your cue to end the session.

Is your baby getting enough milk?

You might be worried that your baby is not be getting enough milk to develop optimally. Here's a couple good ways to tell:

Check his diapers. Pay attention to how many times your baby is peeing and pooping. Newborns typically pee 8-12 times per day. Their urine is typically clear or a very pale yellow. For bowel movements, five is a good average. For the first few weeks, it can be helpful to write down both the breastfeeding session frequency and the diaper output.

Weight. Healthy babies should be gaining weight steadily: the typical newborn gains 2/3 to 1 ounce per day during the first month. From 1 to 4 months babies usually gain 1 ½ to 2 pounds per week. By 6 months, most healthy babies have doubled their birth weight. By the time they reach their first year, your child should have tripled his birth weight.

Important things to know when formula feeding

Washing feeding equipment. It's not necessary to boil or sterilize bottles and artificial nipples if you're washing them thoroughly with warm and clean water. Always remember to clean out any leftovers from the last feeding session, which can always spoil easily and upset your child's digestion.

Throwing out prepared formula. You can store prepared formula in the refrigerator for 48 hrs, but only if the baby hasn't touched the nipple. If he does touch it, get rid of whatever remains after a feeding sesion.

Heating the formula. It's not recommended to heat the formula in the microwave, as microwaves tend to heat unevenly, and hotspots may burn your child. Put the bottle inside a bowl of warm water for a few minutes instead.

Switching up the formula. Sometimes it might be necessary to switch the formula to help settle digestive problems. Switching to a soy formula may help out with some allergic reactions for example, but seek advice from your paediatrician before doing any changes.

Reminders and Safeguards

Holding your child during feedings. Avoid propping your baby up with his bottle - it presents a choking hazard.

Checking your baby's diapers. Your baby's diapers give you a lot of information about how his body is managing new foods. In case your baby seems to become wetting less diapers than normal, call your doctor. Your child might be dehydrated or undernourished.

Find the right nipple hole size. If it's too big, your baby's gag reflex may kick in as he won't know what to do about the fast milk flow. If you notice him struggling, the opening might be not big enough or the nipple might be too hard for him.

Formula feeding

Although nothing truly duplicates the nourishing properties of breast milk, modern formulas can be great for your child. If you opt to supplement breastfeeding, attempt to wait until your child is three or four days old so that your milk supply is well-established.

The moments when you are feeding your child with a bottle are excellent occasions to bond with him and to get to know one each other better. Bottle feeding can be a great way for fathers or other family members to start developing a good relationship with the baby.

A key thing to remember whens when formula feeding is to hold the baby's head at a moderately elevated angle and to hold the bottle up in a way that it prevents him from sucking in air.

Selecting the best formula for your baby

Infant formulas are developed to meet the essential nutritional needs of babies, and try to model the same properties of breast milk. Most formulas contain modified cows' milk, and the standard brands share a lot of similarities. Unless of course your paediatrician tells you otherwise, pick one that includes iron.

Formulas are typically available in three kinds of presentations: ready-to-feed (usually the most expensive), liquid concentrate (less costly), and powder form (which is usually the cheapest).

Following your Baby's Lead

Remember, each baby has his own needs and can vary his required intake from one feeding session to the next. Never pressure-feed him extra formula, and do not leave him smacking his lips wanting more. If your baby spits up frequently, he may do better with smaller sized but more frequent feedings.

Chapter 5: Your baby's development

From defenseless new-born to active toddler: Your baby will only need 12 months to go through this fascinating transformation. Babies develop at an astounding pace, and each month brings exciting and new things for them and their parents.

New parents frequently question what to anticipate next and also wonder about what's the best way to determine if their baby's development is on the right track. Rather than turning all your attention on developmental milestones, it's best to remember that babies all develop at their own pace. There is a fairly wide "window" for when it's normal for any baby to get to a certain milestone.

It's very normal for your child to reach a milestone before expected, and then experience a delay when reaching the next one. This is usually because babies tend to be busy perfecting a skill, and don't like to spend their energy and effort trying out new things. Some babies may say their first word at eight months, while some won't say anything until at least 12 months have gone by. And walking may begin anytime between 9 and 17 months.

Keeping in mind those wide developmental windows, here's what your child might be doing during each important stage of his first year of life.

1 to 3 months

In this first development stage, babies' physiques and brains are learning to take in the outside world. Between birth and three several weeks, your child may begin to:

-Smile. In the earliest stages, he'll be smiling to himself a lot. But within 2-3 months, you'll notice him smiling back in response to your own smiles, and will constantly try to get you to smile back at him.

-When lying on his tummy, he might start raising his head and chest.

-Track objects and movement with his eyes. Eye crossing will steadily decrease.

-Open and close the hands and bring them close to the face.

-Lightly grip objects.

-Take swipes at or try to reach objects nearby, especially those that have a bit of movement and get his attention a lot.

4 to 6 months

Starting from their 4th month, most babies begin to learn and understand how to reach out and manipulate the environment around them. They're becoming more skilled at using their hands. And they're exploring their voices a lot. At this stage, your child will most likely:

-Be able to rollover from front to back and back to front.

-Babble, and make some sounds that resemble language.

-Laugh.

-Reach out and grab stuff (your hair will be constantly pulled!), and play with toys along with other objects using his hands.

-Sit up with some effort and have better control of his head.

7 to 9 months

Throughout the other half of the year, your child will start using his feet and hands a lot more to move. They will also start rolling over a lot! He'll spend a lot of time working out how he can move forwards or backwards on his own. In case you haven't baby-proofed your house yet, now is the time!

At this stage, your child may:

-Begin to crawl. He may also scoot (move while lying on his tummy) or do some "soldier crawling" (dragging himself around on his tummy using the arms and legs), in addition to standard crawling on hands and knees. Some babies never crawl, and transition directly from scooting to walking.

-Sit without any support.

-React to familiar words and sounds such as his name. He might also react to "No" by briefly stopping whatever he was doing and look at you.

-Clap and play simple games with you.

-Pull up to a standing position.

10 to 12 months

The final development stage in your child's first year packs quite a punch. He isn't a baby any more, and will start to develop some habits closely associated to toddlers. But he's still your baby in lots of ways. At this point, he's learning how to:

-Feed himself. Babies at this stage learn how to use their thumbs and index fingers to hold small objects.

-Walk around the room using a bit of support.

-Say a couple of words, such as the classic "Mama" and "Dada", which are specifically designated to each parent. On average, they speak three spoken words when they reach their first birthday, but the range is extremely wide. Some kids say their first words until much later.

-Point at objects he's interested in.

-Mimic your actions and do a bit of "pretend play" by copying things that he usually sees you doing on a regular basis, such as talking on the phone.

Throwing out the pacifier

Sucking on a pacifier has a few benefits for babies, such as soothing them and lowering the risk of sudden infant death syndrome (although it's still a bit of a mystery why). However, after the sixth month, pacifiers become less useful and can be a difficult habit to break. Most paediatricians recommend to wean your baby from the pacifier before he reaches his first year.

There is no clear evidence that pacifiers cause permanent harm to baby teeth - as they often shift back to place after not using one for a few months. However, pacifiers can cause long-term damage to permanent teeth, which start arriving around age four to six. Prolonged pacifier use may cause your son or daughter's upper teeth to tip forward toward the lip, resulting in dental issues. It's very important that your child has completely stopped using one by then.

When it's time to wean your child from the pacifier, do it steadily. Many parents think it is easiest to begin by restricting daytime use, and then begin to cut back on night time use. Beginning a brand new bed time ritual might help too.

When to speak to a doctor.

If your child isn't meeting some important growth or developmental milestones, it is a good idea to trust your instincts. If you feel there's something wrong, talk to your paediatrician about your concerns so that you catch any issues as soon as possible. Early intervention is better, and you know your baby better than anybody.

Remember, that it's not important to pay so much attention on when exactly your baby starts crawling or scooting or saying his first words; it's the fact that he's steadily moving forward through his development stages that really matters. Your baby's development isn't a race, and there's no school application when your baby first crawled or said his first word.

Helping your baby progress

All type of developmental delays can be concerning and cause their own set of issues. For example, language delays can be problematic to a child's academic development. If you notice severe language delays by the time your baby is 2 years old, it's best to get an evaluation.

However, parents can help promote their babies development in several ways:

Gross motor skills

-Place your baby on his tummy more often while he's awake, as it will encourage him to start using more his neck and back muscles.

-Make sure that your home is safe so that your baby can spend more time in the floor and develop his tiny muscles.

-Older babies that can already walk should be spending more time outside.

Fine motor skills

-Give your baby a variety of different toys with interesting textures that will encourage him to explore with their hands more.

-Provide him with age appropriate games, puzzles and colouring materials

- If your baby is capable of feeding himself, encourage him to do it more often.

Language

- Play music often to stimulate his hearing.

- Talk to him more often.

- Read him picture books and name objects as you point them out.

Social interaction

- Avoid leaving him off by himself often.

- Engage with him on a daily basis.

- Laugh and smile with your child.

-Limit TV time and play with him more often.

-Encourage interaction with others you trust.

Conclusion

I hope this book was able to help you gain a better understanding of what to expect from your baby's first year and how to help him transition into a happy and healthy toddler.

Though most parents make lots of mistakes in the 18 years it takes to raise a child; love, attention, and care will always provide strong support for healthy development.

There is no such thing as "too much information" when it comes to raising a child, so make an effort to learn as much as you can from trusted sources and from people who are already a long way down the road you are traveling now.

CPSIA information can be obtained
at www.ICGtesting.com
Printed in the USA
LVHW052156030321
680488LV00015B/151